THE ULTIMATE SLEEP GUIDE

THE ULTIMATE SLEEP GUIDE

DON COLBERT, MD

SILOAM

Most CHARISMA HOUSE BOOK GROUP products are available at special quantity discounts for bulk purchase for sales promotions, premiums, fund-raising, and educational needs. For details, write Charisma House Book Group, 600 Rinehart Road, Lake Mary, Florida 32746, or telephone (407) 333-0600.

THE ULTIMATE SLEEP GUIDE by Don Colbert
Published by Siloam
Charisma Media/Charisma House Book Group
600 Rinehart Road
Lake Mary, Florida 32746
www.charismahouse.com

Cover design by Vincent Pirozzi
Design Director: Justin Evans

Visit the author's website at http://www.drcolbert.com/.

Library of Congress Cataloging-in-Publication Data
Colbert, Don.
  The ultimate sleep guide / Don Colbert. -- First edition.
     pages cm
  Includes bibliographical references.
  ISBN 978-1-62998-188-8 (trade paper) -- ISBN (invalid) 978-1-62998-258-8 (e-book)
  1. Sleep disorders--Popular works. 2. Sleep--Popular works. I. Title.
  RC547.C655 2015
  616.8'498--dc23
                                    2015002708

15 16 17 18 19 — 9 8 7 6 5 4 3 2 1
Printed in the United States of America

CONTENTS

Introduction

THE RED BULL GENERATION

W E LIVE IN a fast-paced society in which nobody seems to have enough time. I call most of my fellow citizens the "too-much bunch."

- They have too much to do.

- They have too little time to do everything.

- They have taken on too much in the way of commitment or responsibility.

- They have too much debt.

- They have too much work to do in any allotted time frame.

- They have too much in the way of clutter and possessions.

- They have too many frustrations and, as a result, may take way too many tranquilizers and stomach medications!

On top of this, we have distorted expectations about what life should be like or should produce.

1

- We expect our children to be perfect...and they are not.

- We expect other people to do the right thing (according to our definition of "right")...and they do not.

- We expect that, while protecting our children from harm and giving them love and guidance, they won't rebel or seek out the very things from which we attempted to protect them.

- We expect our careers to be fulfilling and rewarding...and they are not.

- We expect our new business ventures to soar...and they fall flat.

- We expect our beloveds to be the perfect spouses...and are surprised to find there is no such thing as a perfect person.

Then, to our distorted expectations, we often add a layer of the competitive spirit—keeping up with the Joneses. We continually compare our level of achievement to that of other people and nearly always find ourselves coming up short in one or more categories of comparison.

If there are two cries voiced by overstressed Americans, they seem to be these:

- "I'm so busy!"

- "I'm so tired!"

Both cries stem from taking on too much to do in too little time.

Anytime I see a patient whose health is deteriorating because life is spinning too fast, I explain to him that life is not a sprint but a marathon. He needs to slow down and enjoy the slow jog through life. Those who race through their days at a breakneck speed are striving—they are in hot pursuit of things temporal that they believe they personally must own, accomplish, or make happen.

In most cases those who are too busy or too tired have a deep intuitive feeling that the one thing they truly need more of is "people time." They need to spend more time with a spouse or with their children. They may need to spend more time with elderly parents, grandchildren, or friends. To get more people time, a person simply needs to turn off some things—for example, the television, the computer, or the phone—and turn on activities that involve conversation, doing tasks together, or engaging in recreational pursuits with other people.

The third great cry I hear from overstressed people is this: "I have too much to do!" Usually this can be translated, "I've taken on too many commitments" or "I'm working too many hours."

What underlies these external factors? Usually a deep desire for more material possessions or a desire for more recognition, fame, or approval. Millions of Americans are living with an excess of possessions and inadequate space. Perhaps they are attempting to buy friendships or feelings of self-worth by taking on too many responsibilities (including participation in a variety of committees, clubs, and societies or care of another person for whom one is not truly responsible).

I have several patients who are "malling" themselves to death—they are addicted to the high they get while shopping and spending, oftentimes, money they truly do not have. The average American now carries the burden of about fifteen thousand dollars in credit card debt,[1] which means our nation as a whole has more than eight hundred billion dollars in credit card debt.[2] Sears now makes more money on credit than it does on the sale of merchandise—and this from a company founded by a man who would only pay cash![3]

THE WALLS COME TUMBLING DOWN

What happens when a very high percentage of our nation is too busy, too tired, and has too much to do for reasons that are often rooted in materialism and striving for self-worth? At least three consequences are directly linked.

1. Relationships suffer.

First, relationships suffer. The divorce rate in our nation has more than doubled since 1950, with approximately one out of every two marriages failing. The majority of new marriages won't last longer than seven years.[4] The one thing that people really need—deeper and more satisfying relationships—is the first thing sacrificed by being too busy, tired, or having too much to do.

2. An obsession with escapism develops.

Second, people become obsessed with new ways to try escaping from the pressures they feel. They seek out more entertainment in the form of books, television programs, videos, video games, and computer games. The average television viewer now watches between twenty and thirty-six hours a week of television.[5]

These people seek out more toys to own, more vacation spots to visit, and more activities or hobbies to help them "unwind." As part of an attempt to escape the pressure, more and more people are eating out or turning to fast-food meals. And what do these various forms of escape produce? In the vast majority of cases, they produce an overwhelming amount of information (far more than a person can take in and use), an overwhelming amount of sexual images (that tend to fuel lust and, eventually, behavior that destroys relationships), an overwhelming amount of expense, and an overwhelmingly unhealthy dietary plan!

3. A distorted view of what is valuable develops.

Third, people who are too tired, too busy, or have too much to do tend to lose sight of what is important because they become preoccupied with what is urgent. They respond to the need of the moment rather than plan and pursue a life that is grounded in what they truly consider to be vital and valuable.

Consider what happens in the workplace. The big goals of doing a job often get bogged down in a sea of cell phone rings, e-mails, voice mails, texts, and instant messages. The average office worker now receives just over one hundred messages from e-mails, memos, and voice mails a day![6]

THIS CYCLE COULD KILL YOU—LITERALLY

It sometimes takes a near-death experience before a person will clarify his values and return to a life structured around self-generated priorities rather than external demands.

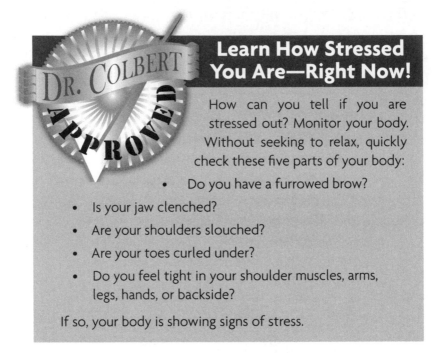

DR. COLBERT APPROVED

Learn How Stressed You Are—Right Now!

How can you tell if you are stressed out? Monitor your body. Without seeking to relax, quickly check these five parts of your body:

- Do you have a furrowed brow?
- Is your jaw clenched?
- Are your shoulders slouched?
- Are your toes curled under?
- Do you feel tight in your shoulder muscles, arms, legs, hands, or backside?

If so, your body is showing signs of stress.

Take the example of a patient of mine named Bill who suffered a massive heart attack in his mid-forties and was not expected to live. His family gathered around his bedside and reminisced with him about the joyful times in their lives. This man had been a highly driven executive who suffered extreme frustration. He sacrificed his family life to climb the corporate ladder. He was closing deals while his children had ball games. He felt driven to succeed.

Bill developed severe hypertension and sky-high cholesterol. He was overweight and had diabetes. His problems compounded at home, to a great extent, because of his absence as a father. His teenage children began experimenting with drugs and eventually became addicted. His son was arrested for drug possession and later for selling Ecstasy and served time in prison. His daughter became an alcoholic and had several abortions. She became so depressed that she tried to commit suicide on a number of occasions. His other son became a homosexual and contracted AIDS. His wife, depressed and overwhelmed, used food for her comfort. She was thin when she married Bill, but her emotional eating made her morbidly obese.

Bill's world was falling apart, literally. His body was broken. The people he loved the most were broken. It was at the time his son was sent to prison that he had his massive heart attack.

Bill defeated all odds and lived through this heart attack, and he made a decision to change his life dramatically. He no longer fought traffic to try to outmaneuver others to reach his destination three minutes earlier. He slowed down, noticed flowers he had never seen in his neighborhood, and took walks in the fresh air. He made a decision that he was truly going to enjoy every day of the rest of his life. He began to write regularly to his son in prison. He reconnected with his daughter and other son and began to attend church with his family every week. He and his wife began to work out at a gym, and they made a mutual decision they were going to stop striving and return to the priorities and goals they had when they first married: a loving, healthy, giving, God-centered marriage.

Did Bill and his wife find instant success in their turn-around efforts? No. But a great deal of pressure lifted from Bill the minute he decided to make these changes.

Are Bill and his wife still in pursuit of the goals and priorities they deeply desire? Yes. Both of them are at greater peace—with far less frustration and striving and stress clouding their days—and they are rebuilding broken relationships with "new bricks" of love, patience, and renewed understanding.

TRUST ME, I GET IT

I've been there, believe me. Lest you think I'm a doctor who only knows how to dispense advice without having lived through what creates the need for that advice in the first place, let me share with you my personal story.

In my third year of medical school, while running a three-mile run in 95-degree weather, with almost 100 percent humidity, I suffered a massive heat stroke. My body temperature reached 108 degrees Fahrenheit.

I was rushed to a hospital emergency room where I received intravenous fluids. My leg muscles were literally bursting—the medical condition is called rhabdomyolysis. I watched as my legs withered before my eyes. The pain was excruciating.

I was hospitalized for two to three weeks so I could receive massive amounts of intravenous fluids and be monitored for kidney failure. I began urinating coffee-colored urine from the muscle breakdown, and I was so weak that I eventually was forced to use a wheelchair.

Rather than improving, my condition grew worse as my leg muscles continued to deteriorate in spite of all the treatments. A surgeon was called in to perform a muscle biopsy. This revealed extensive muscle necrosis—in other words, muscle cell death. I was told I would probably never walk again. By this time my arms actually appeared larger than my legs.

I felt under extreme stress. I had missed more than a month of medical school, and now I was being told I would probably never walk again!

I needed a miracle, and I received one. After a couple of months of rest and a lot of prayer, I was able to walk again. Miraculously I regained the strength as well as the size of my leg muscles.

But as a result of missing so much school, I had a significant amount of makeup work to do. Medical school is difficult enough without falling a month behind. Again, prayer and God's wisdom about how best to use my time and focus on my studies pulled me through.

But then after I graduated from medical school, I began my internship and residency at Florida Hospital in Orlando, Florida, in the specialty of family medicine. I was on call every fourth night and usually did not sleep while on call. The stress of a resident's schedule and the demands of the work—which often are stressful to the point that many medical school graduates burn out during this period—were compounded by the birth of our son, Kyle. I pressed on, however!

In my second year of residency I worked part-time or moonlighted in emergency rooms one to two weekends a month. One emergency room had a forty-eight-hour shift over the weekend. That was a particularly rough job since I got no sleep all weekend and then had to be present bright and early for my training as a resident on Monday morning.

After residency I opened a solo private practice in family medicine. I worked five days a week and took "beeper call" every night for years. I did not take a vacation for ten years. Many nights I was awakened from a sound sleep by patients who called with rather minor problems, such as constipation or insomnia. One couple actually phoned to ask me to give them some marriage counseling by phone at four o'clock in the morning!

I had increased irritability and fatigue, and it became more and more difficult to concentrate. I also became more forgetful. Some mornings my wife would ask me who had called in the middle of the night and awakened us, and I would look at her with uncertainty on my face. I had actually forgotten who had called and whether or not I had phoned in a prescription and even what the prescription was. Research now shows that just one sleepless night can impair driving performance as much as an alcohol blood level of 0.10 percent, which is higher than the legal limit for driving.[7]

I literally became so fatigued keeping up with this lifestyle that I had to put my car in park when I stopped at a red light because I feared I would fall asleep at the light. I would even fall asleep shortly after a movie would start, even though I would really want to see the movie. I would also nearly fall asleep on a forty-minute drive to the beach even with my wife talking to me. I was truly sleep deprived.

The stress of this pace eventually took its toll on my body, as well as on my mind and emotions. One morning I awakened with intense itching and a rash on my legs. I applied hydrocortisone cream, but the rash and itching worsened and spread to my knees, arms, elbows, and hands. I thought I might have contracted scabies from a patient I had seen recently. I applied Kwell lotion from my chin down, but the rash and itching grew worse.

Finally I consulted a dermatologist—a friend of mine—and he diagnosed me as having psoriasis, but not the typical psoriasis with plaques and silvery scales. He prescribed cold tar creams that caused me to smell like kerosene and stained my clothes and sheets yellow orange. The rash and itching persisted.

DR. COLBERT APPROVED

Are You Exhausted? A Test for Adrenal Exhaustion

If you feel dizzy or lightheaded when you stand up suddenly, it may be an indicator that you are in the exhaustion stage of stress.

A simple screening test for adrenal exhaustion is to have your blood pressure checked while lying down. Rest for five minutes. Then stand up and immediately have your blood pressure checked again. If it drops by ten points, it's very likely that your adrenals are exhausted. Just be sure that you are not dehydrated, because that can produce the same effect.

I test patients' adrenal function by checking salivary cortisol levels at 8:00 a.m., noon, 4:00 p.m., and 8:00 p.m. I also check DHEA sulfate levels.

Many of my patients took one look at my skin and asked me about my "problem." They no doubt feared I was contagious!

Eventually, through detoxification procedures and nutritional supplementation, the psoriasis cleared up, but I began to notice that it would flare up again every time I was severely stressed.

The stress of excessive work—not only the long hours and pressures associated with medicine, but also too many nights on call without any breaks—caused me to feel extremely fatigued, and my immune system became compromised. I developed recurrent sinus infections and took antibiotics frequently to treat the sinusitis. Then I developed severe irritable bowel syndrome, with abdominal pain, bloating, and episodes of diarrhea. The tremendous fatigue led to short-term memory loss.

To top it all off, I continued to feel overwhelmed emotionally by the debt I had incurred in opening up a solo private practice while paying off medical-school loans. Like many physicians I also feared potential lawsuits and found the rising costs of malpractice insurance to be a staggering financial burden. In other words, I was also suffering from anxiety.

All of these factors seemed to influence one another to create something of a downward spiral—the fatigue grew worse; my immune system was further weakened; and the chronic sinusitis, psoriasis, and irritable bowel syndrome were aggravated.

The more I suffered from infections and irritable bowel syndrome, the more fatigue I felt and the weaker my immune system became. I was trapped! I was a medical doctor, but I was sick—I was literally stewing in my own juices and saw no way out of my predicament.

I remember what a psychiatry professor—a former dermatologist—shared during a lecture in medical school. In his previous practice he treated many patients who had suffered with psoriasis. I was curious as to why he no longer practiced as a dermatologist but instead chose psychiatry, and his answer surprised me. He told me that treating so many people suffering from skin disorders led him to the conclusion that people were actually "weeping through their skin." That is what prompted him to go back to residency training in psychiatry. He knew the skin disorder was just a superficial sign of a much deeper problem.

That should have been the time when things hit

bottom...but no. I compounded my own stress by writing books and facing publisher deadlines. By then my son had become a teenager and went through a rebellious stage. I spent many sleepless nights in prayer for him.

In search of answers for my own health problems, I spent the next few years learning nutrition, detoxification, and a healthy diet, as well as the importance of stress reduction and dealing with deadly emotions. However, I did not regain my health until I began getting adequate restorative sleep, repaying the sleep debt I had accrued, and living a more restful life.

You see, lack of true rest had impaired my alertness, work performance, concentration, and memory, and I eventually lost my health from lack of sleep. Here I was, only in my early thirties, and I had sacrificed my health by choosing to be on call and not paying attention to the warning signs my body and mind were giving me.

Finally, I woke up to the fact that my main problem was lack of adequate rest, and I then began to share calls with other physicians. Eventually I stopped taking night calls altogether. Making sleep a priority—going to bed at about the same time each night, waking up at about the same time each morning, and not being awakened during the night—enabled me to repay the tremendous sleep debt that I had accumulated and thus regain my health.

YOU CAN REST IN THIS

Do I know about the rat race, about striving to keep up, about moving through life without adequate rest, about not knowing how to escape the unending cycle? Indeed, I do.

I had to learn to deal with a lack of adequate rest—not

in theory, but in order to survive. The information you will read in this book is what I applied to my own life. It literally saved me from mental, emotional, and physical illness, and probably an early death. I continue to live by these principles, which I have also taught to countless other people. I count it a privilege to share these truths with you.

If I could find a way out of my own "energy drink" approach to life and have helped others, like Bill, find their way out, I have no doubt that you can too. You do not have to keep up with the Joneses, drag yourself through exhausted days, or suffer through sleepless nights. It's possible to start right now on a new life plan—one that fills your life with buoyant vitality rooted in a restful way of life.

The truth is, God never intended for you to push through your days and months feeling increasingly weary. Jesus said:

> Come to me, all of you who are weary and carry heavy burdens, and I will give you rest. Take my yoke upon you. Let me teach you, because I am humble and gentle at heart, and you will find rest for your souls. For my yoke is easy to bear, and the burden I give you is light.
> —MATTHEW 11:28–30, NLT

If your current pace of life has left you feeling exhausted, depleted, and defeated, rest assured that these things are not God's will for you. If you are struggling to find balance and rest, there's hope! Let's discover that hope together—starting with the reason good rest is so vital to our health.

z Building Blocks to a Better z Night's Sleep

- Be honest with yourself—what's the shape of your personal rat race at the moment? What's the real cost of what you're striving to get or achieve?

- Know that eventually the toll will reveal itself. Your relationships will suffer, you'll go into escape mode, and you'll lose sight of what really matters. Have you reached that point? Are you ready to cash in your chips yet?

- You do not have to keep up with the Joneses, drag yourself through exhausted days, or suffer through sleepless nights. God wants something infinitely better for you—and it begins with adequate rest.

Chapter 1

WHY DO I NEED TO SLEEP?

W HEN PRESIDENT CLINTON first ran for the presidency, he declared that he went the last forty-eight hours of his campaign without sleep because of his passion to become president.[1] But later, after a series of scandals, Clinton changed his mind about sleep. He said that every important mistake he had made in his life, he made because he was too tired. In fact, former White House counsel Beth Nolan blamed one Clinton-era scandal on sleep deprivation. She told Congress that she had been going on a couple of hours of sleep most nights that week, as had the president. "Had I been operating on more sleep, had the president been operating on more sleep...there would have been more calls made," she said.[2]

Many professions in today's stressed-out world create fatigue and encourage sleep deprivation. It is believed that a century ago, before Thomas Edison invented the light bulb, the average person slept about ten hours per night. Today the average individual sleeps less than seven hours a night.[3] We live in a world where day and night no longer matter. Thanks to modern technology we can work and play around the clock. What's more, our modern lifestyles are so full that there's usually not enough time to get everything done, and consequently we tend to short ourselves on sleep. We end up paying for our many activities with drowsiness and fatigue.

I see the evidence in my medical practice. The number one complaint I hear from patients who come into my office is, "I'm tired." They slump forward in their chairs, peering at me from under the weight of fatigue. I fear to send some of them out of my office because they don't seem awake enough to drive home!

This is not the way our bodies or minds were made to operate. God gave us a promise of deep, restorative sleep. Psalm 127:2 (NKJV) says, "He gives His beloved sleep." God wants so much more for you than this, and if you take the guidance in this book to heart, you can be on your way to life as God meant you to know it.

SOUND THE ALARM

Let's begin by taking a look at a few statistics related to our growing problem with sleep.

- A 2005 survey by the National Sleep Foundation found 75 percent of adults had at least one symptom of a sleep problem, and 54 percent experienced at least one symptom of insomnia.[4]

- Americans average a little less than seven hours of sleep a night, but sleep experts generally recommend seven to eight hours of sleep a night.[5]

- Approximately 40 percent of adults snore.[6]

- Approximately 60 percent of children, mainly teenagers, report being tired during the day.[7]

- Women suffer from insomnia more often than men.[8]

- As men go from sixteen years of age to fifty years of age, they lose about 80 percent of their deep sleep, according to one study.[9]

- Insomnia is more common in people over the age of sixty-five, with more than half of those over age sixty-five experiencing disturbed sleep.[10]

- Elderly people also commonly take different prescription medications, with insomnia being one of the side effects.[11]

- Elderly people are also more prone to develop anxiety, depression, and grief, which are associated with insomnia.[12]

- Of all adults, 20 to 40 percent have insomnia in the course of a year.[13]

- Over seventy million Americans suffer from disorders of sleep and wakefulness.[14]

- One out of three people have insomnia at some point in their lives.[15]

- Insomnia is the third most frequent health complaint behind headaches (the second) and pain (first).[16]

- People with insomnia are more prone to develop depression.[17]

- An estimated fifty to seventy million Americans live on the brink of mental and physical collapse because of lack of sleep.[18]

- Researchers found that in one year alone, about forty-two million sleeping pill prescriptions were filled for American adults and children.[19]

- An estimated 60 million Americans suffer from insomnia and other sleep disorders.[20]

- More than half of all American adults suffer from insomnia at least a few times each week. As a result, over 50 percent of the American population will experience daytime drowsiness.[21]

- Evidence suggests inadequate rest and sleep may shorten life span by eight to ten years.[22]

- A recent survey revealed that approximately 40 percent of all adults claimed they were so drowsy that it interfered with their daily activities.[23]

- More than half of the American adult population experiences drowsiness during the day.[24]

These statistics are staggering—but that's not even the whole of it. The medical research is clear about what happens when you don't get sufficient sleep.

1. You increase your risk of developing type 2 diabetes.
One study published by the medical journal *Lancet* revealed that even in young, healthy individuals, a sleep deficit of three

to four hours a night over the course of a week affected the body's ability to process carbohydrates, leading some people into a prediabetic state.[25] Furthermore, one study found that people who limited their sleep to only four hours a night for several nights experienced changes in hormones that control appetite, resulting in overeating and weight gain,[26] demonstrating that a lack of adequate sleep puts you at a greater risk for obesity.

2. You increase your risk of heart disease.

A 2004 study found that women who averaged only five hours of sleep a night were 39 percent more likely to develop heart disease than those who slept eight hours a night.[27]

3. You become clumsy and "sleep drunk."

Lack of sleep slows your reaction time, shortens your attention span, and impairs your memory, your decision-making process, and your coordination. People who go for up to nineteen hours without sleep score significantly worse on performance and alertness tests than people with a blood alcohol level of .08, which is legally drunk.[28]

4. You jeopardize your job.

According to the National Commission on Sleep Disorders at the National Institutes of Health in Bethesda, Maryland, sleep deprivation costs an estimated $150 billion a year in higher stress and reduced workplace productivity.[29]

A third of America's adult workers either missed work or made mistakes at work in the past three months because of a lack of sleep.[30] Nobody drinks on the job, but plenty of people come to work after pulling all-nighters or getting too little sleep, thus functioning as if they were drunk.

5. You endanger your life and the lives of others.

Sleep deprivation is responsible for at least one hundred thousand crashes and fifteen hundred fatalities a year, according to a 2002 report from the National Highway Traffic Safety Administration. Half of Americans admit to driving while drowsy. Studies show huge peaks in the number of accidents caused by people falling asleep at the wheel in the middle of the night and smaller peaks in the middle of the afternoon.[31]

6. You reduce your sex drive.

Sleep deprivation raises cortisol levels, which blocks the normal response of the testicles to testosterone and decreases the production of hormonal precursors to testosterone. This is one reason young men in military boot camp generally have a lower sex drive, believe it or not.[32]

7. You invite diseases.

A host of physical conditions are associated with insomnia, including chronic fatigue, fibromyalgia, chronic pain syndrome, autoimmune diseases, hypertension, obesity, depression, and other forms of mental illness.

Adults with commonly diagnosed health conditions such as high blood pressure, arthritis, heartburn, and depression say they rarely get a good night's sleep, showing an association between sleeplessness and disease. People with these conditions are nearly twice as likely to experience frequent daytime sleepiness as those who don't have the conditions.[33]

8. You jeopardize your marriage.

Studies show higher rates of divorce among people who don't get adequate sleep.[34] Getting the adequate amount of sleep is beneficial to you, and it benefits those around you.

9. You create many more problems.

Here's a further rundown of what you risk if you don't get enough rest:

- Loss of focus, concentration, memory, and creativity, as well as alertness and work performance

- Problems making decisions

- Less opportunity to recharge, restore, and refresh your brain and body

- Imbalanced neurotransmitters such as serotonin, norepinephrine, and dopamine, which are commonly associated with anxiety, depression, irritability, grumpiness, and mood swings

- Compromised immune system and decreased number of natural killer cells, resulting in more colds, flu, and other infections.

- Increased risk of cancer due to lower natural-killer-cell count and a weaker immune system

- Higher risk of inflammation, which is at the root of most degenerative diseases—including heart disease, cancer, Alzheimer's disease, arthritis, asthma, and many more diseases

- Increased headaches, sore joints, and stomach ailments

UNDERSTANDING SLEEP DEBT

As I mentioned in this book's introduction, I suffered tremendous sleep deprivation during my medical residency and early years of practice. I was on call every fourth night. I often went through the night without sleeping and then had to work the following day. During that season of my life I felt fatigued and drowsy much of the time.

The truth is, the less sleep we get, the more we build up sleep debt, and it can be hard to catch up. The health problems I experienced in my thirties were the result of accumulating a huge sleep debt. My body needed a certain amount of sleep per night in order to function at its best. Typically I need at least eight hours sleep a night in order to function at my best. Instead of getting eight hours of sleep a night during internship and residency, I would only get about one to two hours of sleep at night every fourth night. So, I would have a six- or seven-hour sleep debt on the nights that I was on call.

The difference between the number of hours that you need to sleep each night—which is about eight hours for me—and the number of hours you actually sleep equal your sleep debt. For example, I was sleeping maybe one hour on Monday, eight hours on Tuesday, eight hours on Wednesday, eight hours on Thursday, and one hour on Friday. Thus, I built up a sleep debt of fourteen hours in just five days.

Now, the greater your sleep debt is, the stronger the drive for sleep. Also, your sleep debt is cumulative. A sleep debt is very similar to someone who regularly withdraws more money from their bank account than they deposit. They get further and further into the red as each day passes.

As another example, my son's last semester of college was quite difficult. He pulled many all-nighters studying and had accumulated a hefty sleep debt as a result. Also, his first baby was born during the middle of all of this. When he returned home from school, he slept about twelve to fourteen hours a night for the first couple of weeks after arriving. I understood this as he was repaying his sleep debt that he owed his body.

As you accumulate more and more sleep debt, fatigue and irritability increase, and job performance, memory, and concentration decrease. You are also at a higher risk of having a traffic accident or job injury, and eventually health problems begin to occur.

YOU CAN ALSO SLEEP TOO MUCH

Just as inadequate sleep is associated with many health problems, too much sleep is also associated with its own set of heath issues. Numerous medical problems are associated with too much sleep, including type 2 diabetes and obesity. In one study of almost nine thousand Americans, people who slept more than nine hours per night had a 50 percent greater risk of diabetes than individuals who slept seven hours per night. An increased risk of diabetes was also seen in those who slept less than five hours per night.[35]

Also, another study showed that individuals who slept for nine or more hours per night were 21 percent more likely to become obese over a six-year period than those who slept between seven and eight hours per night.[36]

Multiple studies have found that those who sleep nine or

more hours per night have a significantly higher death rate than those sleeping seven to eight hours a night.[37]

Researchers have found that in postmenopausal women, those who slept nine or more hours per night were 70 percent more likely to suffer an ischemic stroke than those females who slept an average of seven hours per night. The females who slept six hours or less per night are at a 14 percent higher risk of stroke compared to those who slept seven hours per night.[38]

However, for those sleeping nine hours a night, they should not think they are going to die early. The best way to determine whether you get enough sleep is by asking yourself two questions:

1. Do you awaken refreshed?

2. Are you alert during the day?

The main thing to understand is that too much sleep can be just as dangerous to your health as inadequate sleep.

RESTORE YOURSELF

Every night when the Walt Disney World theme parks close their gates and the crowds go home, the most important hours of the Disney day begin. Big lights go up, and massive crews of workers repair and clean every ride, every walkway, and every concession stand. When the gates open the next morning, the parks are completely renewed. The trash from the previous day is gone, and the roller coasters are in top condition again.

A similar thing happens every night in your body. During

those precious hours your body shuts down and repairs itself. Your immune system recharges. Your major organs are restored. Old cells are being replaced with new ones. Your mind relaxes and orders its thoughts, creating a healthy mental state.

But what if Walt Disney World stayed open all night or let people in at 3:00 a.m., cutting short the repair time? The park would eventually be unsafe, unsanitary, and unappealing. It would end up a run-down shadow of itself, careening toward financial disaster and, worse, causing injuries or deaths on rides that were not maintained properly.

Lack of sleep is just as disastrous for you as an individual. A good night's sleep is free. A bad night's sleep is costly, because it takes a toll on your health. Sleep and rest are so important because of what they do for your health.

Here are just a handful of ways good rest restores you.

1. Sleep regulates release of important hormones.

When you sleep, growth hormone is secreted. This causes children to grow, and it regulates muscle mass and helps control fat in adults. When you don't sleep enough, this hormone's function is disrupted. Perhaps lack of sleep is partially to blame for the fact that two-thirds of Americans are overweight or obese. Leptin, another hormone, is secreted during sleep and directly influences appetite and weight control. It tells the body when it is "full." A person who doesn't have enough of this regulating hormone often has a runaway appetite.

2. Sleep slows the aging process.

The term *beauty rest* is literally true. Growth hormone is mainly secreted at night as we sleep, along with other hormones that help to keep us looking younger. Sleep slows the aging process, and some say it is one of the most important "secrets" for averting wrinkles. How well a person sleeps is one of the most important predictors of how long a person will live.

3. Sleep boosts the immune system.

People who sleep nine hours a night instead of seven hours have greater than normal "natural killer cell" activity. Natural killer cells destroy viruses, bacteria, and cancer cells.

4. Sleep improves brain function.

One study shows that short-term sleep deprivation may decrease brain activity related to alertness and cognitive performance.[39]

5. Sleep reduces cortisol levels.

Excessive stress raises cortisol levels, which disrupt neurotransmitter balance in the brain, causing you to be more irritable and prone to depression, anxiety, and insomnia. High cortisol levels are associated with many diseases, but the cure is as close as your pillow. Sufficient sleep helps to reduce cortisol levels.

Good sleep is one of the best "health principles" available to you, and yet relatively few people get adequate sleep. As a society, Americans are chronically sleep deprived. One in six claim that insomnia is a major problem for them. By not sleeping, they degrade and even ruin their health.[40]

THE EVIDENCE IS IN

Simply put, the benefits to your body and mind of plenty of restful sleep cannot be measured. Sleep is absolutely vital to your health and well-being. During sleep you recharge your mind and body. Sleep allows your body to recuperate and restore itself from exhaustion. In addition, during sleep your cells are able to regenerate and rejuvenate because the body secretes growth hormones as you slumber that signal it to repair tissues and organs.

Sleep gives your mind a mental break, and it helps to restore your memory. Dreaming helps your mind to sort out and resolve emotional conflicts. During sleep your body rebuilds and removes toxins. As you rest your body mentally and physically, your energy is increased.

We spend up to one-third of our lives asleep, so getting adequate rest is critical for our health. Without enough sleep the body begins to degenerate more rapidly. Adequate sleep actually helps to lower cortisol, the stress hormone. If our brains are deprived of sleep over the long term, brain aging results.

Sleep deprivation and excessive fatigue can also lead to anxiety, depression, and extreme irritability, and they can cause you to gain weight. Lack of sleep can dramatically undermine your immune system, which leads to more colds, flus, and other infectious diseases.

Fatigue will also lead to impaired mental function, causing problems at work or at school. The sleep-deprived tend to be more forgetful and less able to concentrate and focus. Decreased eye/hand coordination can result in a higher incidence of accidents and motor vehicle accidents.

Almighty God, who created the universe with unparalleled wisdom, also created your body to need rest. As a matter of fact, in His wisdom God made rest a foundational principle for life on Earth. The Bible says, "And on the seventh day

God ended His work which He had done, and He rested on the seventh day from all His work which He had done. Then God blessed the seventh day and sanctified it, because in it He rested from all His work which God had created and made" (Gen. 2:2–3). Rest is a gift to all the earth's creatures to restore and refresh their physical, mental, and spiritual strength and to renew their vitality.

The rest your body needs is a vital part of living in God's divine health for you, and your loving Creator is committed to seeing that you get it. Take a moment and think about the heavenly Father's heart as you read these words: "The LORD is my shepherd, I shall not want. He makes me lie down in green pastures; He leads me beside quiet waters. He restores my soul" (Ps. 23:1–3, NAS).

If you are suffering because of not getting enough sleep, rest assured. God has provided wisdom to help you to gain a better understanding of the reasons for your fatigue so that you can begin feeling much better very soon.

Building Blocks to a Better Night's Sleep

- The health risks of insufficient rest are almost too numerous to count—type 2 diabetes, heart disease, cancer, obesity, accidents. The list goes on and on.

- The health benefits of a lifestyle of rest, on the other hand, are vast. You can slow down your aging, enjoy a greater quality of life, improve your immune system and brain function—to name but a few!

- Sleep debt is real, and you don't want to fall behind. Furthermore, sleeping too much carries its own fair share of risks. Aim for seven to nine hours of sleep per night consistently.

Chapter 2

THE ARCHITECTURE OF SLEEP

M ANY PEOPLE IN everyday life brag that they only need four or five hours of sleep a night. It's usually the same people who chug energy drinks, such as Red Bull, and pop energy pills for breakfast. Anyone who thinks they are getting the most out of life with just a few hours of sleep is kidding himself. It means, rather, that he has learned to function at a much lower level of mental and physical capacity, sustained artificially and temporarily by the adrenal glands and his caffeinated drink of choice.

We need to recognize that God designed our bodies to need sleep. We need this downtime every night to restore, remove, and replace worn-out and dead cells in the body. We also need adequate sleep to give the brain an opportunity to sort out the information of the day in ways that are intricately designed by our Creator and are far too complex to begin to explain here. In extremely simplified terms, we need a sufficient break from sensory input in order to categorize and store information for use as memories that guide future behavior.

As part of recognizing that we need sleep, we must come to value sleep. A majority of Americans, however, don't seem to value sleep enough to get the sleep they need. During times of illness or stress, you may typically feel an increased need for sleep. Unfortunately for most Americans, when they are pressed for time or are working to meet a deadline, the first thing they usually cut back on is sleep. One thing you need to realize is that adequate sleep is not an option or a luxury but a major component of good health.

How Much Sleep Do You Need?

Sleep needs vary from person to person. However, most sleep experts recommend that adults get seven to eight hours of restful sleep per night; people who practice this tend to be the healthiest. Then there's the fact that the amount of sleep you need will vary over the course of your life and is dependent on your age, activity level, stress level, health, as well as lifestyle habits.

A well-known minister who is a good friend of mine told me, "Before I heard your teaching on sleep, I thought I could live on six hours of sleep a day. Now I wake up early, look at my watch, and think, 'Hmm. I've got to lie here for two more hours.' But I feel more refreshed. My mind is clearer."

Many patients come into my office complaining of fatigue and tell me they get six or seven hours of sleep a night. I give them the cell phone analogy. Your phone won't last as long if you don't totally recharge it. These people, like their gadgets, run out of energy in the middle of the day.

Most adults need seven to nine hours of sleep a night without interruption. Infants need more—about fourteen hours a day.[1] A five-year-old needs twelve hours a day. Most people find that eight hours is perfect. Any less and you feel drowsy at some point during the day. Any more and you may feel unnaturally sluggish.

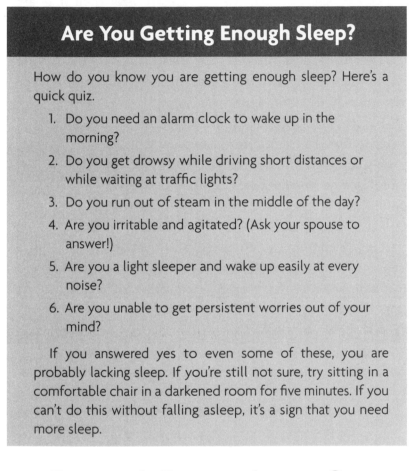

Are You Getting Enough Sleep?

How do you know you are getting enough sleep? Here's a quick quiz.

1. Do you need an alarm clock to wake up in the morning?
2. Do you get drowsy while driving short distances or while waiting at traffic lights?
3. Do you run out of steam in the middle of the day?
4. Are you irritable and agitated? (Ask your spouse to answer!)
5. Are you a light sleeper and wake up easily at every noise?
6. Are you unable to get persistent worries out of your mind?

If you answered yes to even some of these, you are probably lacking sleep. If you're still not sure, try sitting in a comfortable chair in a darkened room for five minutes. If you can't do this without falling asleep, it's a sign that you need more sleep.

BREAKING IT DOWN BY AGE AND STAGE

As I've stated, most adults require seven to eight hours of sleep a night; however, we did not start off that way. As newborns, we slept approximately twelve to eighteen hours a day and did not adhere to a schedule. However, by six months of age most infants are able to sleep through the night for about nine to twelve hours and usually take a nap in the morning and afternoon for thirty minutes to two hours.

Toddlers, ages one to three years of age, sleep approximately twelve to fourteen hours a night with just one nap during the day for approximately one to three hours.

Preschoolers, ages three to five, sleep about eleven to thirteen hours a night, and naps are usually shorter. After age five, most children no longer need a nap.

Children six years of age to puberty usually sleep about ten to eleven hours a night. Their sleep patterns are very similar to the sleep pattern of adults.

Adolescents usually need about nine to ten hours of sleep per night, but they usually do not attain it and begin to develop a sleep debt.

After age sixty most adults still need seven to eight hours sleep a night in order to be refreshed and alert. However, most elderly people have problems getting adequate sleep at night.

Elderly individuals need to realize that their overall health is directly associated with good sleep quality as well as an adequate amount of sleep.

ALL THE STAGES OF SLEEP

It's not just the length of sleep that matters, but also the depth of sleep and the number of cycles you go through. Normal sleep occurs in cycles, with most people experiencing five to six sleep cycles during a normal night. Each cycle lasts sixty to ninety minutes and has two parts, with the first part including four stages and the second part including one stage.

The two main parts of sleep are:

- Non–rapid eye movement (NREM) sleep. NREM is a cycle with four stages: stage one, stage two, stage three, and stage four, with stage four being the deepest sleep. When you close your eyes and doze off, stage one begins.

- Rapid eye movement (REM) sleep. By the time you've entered stage five, you've moved into REM sleep. This is the level of sleep where dreaming takes place. During REM sleep the brain is very active.

Completing a sleep cycle means that you've drifted from being in superficial stage one sleep all the way through stages two and three, and then you entered stage four, your deepest sleep. After that, you entered stage five, which is the dream stage.

Here is what happens in each stage:

- Stage one sleep is the drowsy stage in which you drift in and out of being awake. During stage one sleep it's easy to be awakened, for you are actually just dozing or are half-awake.

- Stage two sleep, on the other hand, is a light level of sleep. Here your heart rate, respiratory rate, and metabolic rate decrease. During stage two you can still be awakened easily.

- Stage three sleep is the level where your breathing slows down. Your heart rate slows even more, and your muscles become more relaxed. During this stage the body is able to regenerate, restore, and repair organs and tissues due to the release of growth hormone. You generally reach stage three sleep within thirty minutes of falling asleep. It's more difficult to awaken someone from stage three sleep. When you do wake them up, they tend to be a little groggy.

• Stage four sleep is the deepest level of sleep, and it is the most restorative and refreshing stage of sleep. This stage is reached approximately an hour after falling asleep, and it is by far the most important stage of sleep. After two to three sleep cycles, both stage three and stage four sleep may disappear for the remainder of the night. That's why it's critically important to get uninterrupted, peaceful, restorative sleep for the first three sleep cycles, which occur during the first four and a half hours of sleep. This is the best way to reap the benefit of this deep, restoring, and repairing stage three and stage four sleep.

• Stage five sleep—the final stage—is REM sleep, also called dream sleep. During REM sleep the brain is much more active as the brain reacts to dreams. In fact, the EEG tracing during REM sleep reveals rapid alpha waves that are very similar to the brain waves present when you are awake. Your heart rate and respiratory rate may speed up a little during REM sleep.

Sleep and dreams play a huge part in your mental health. REM sleep is responsible for memory consolidation. During sleep our brains take different memories and examine how well they fit or don't fit together. Dreams serve to bring mysterious images from the unconscious soul to the wakeful consciousness where we can lay them out in front of us, examine them, dissect them, and glean meaning from them. These images often reflect issues we need to address in order to become whole. There are many biblical examples of how God used dreams to make people aware of important matters in their world and to help them prepare solutions to forthcoming challenges. Today, dreams can serve the same purpose for us. They connect us with our internal intelligence, our true selves, and our souls. They are images that have the ability to bring wellness and wholeness.

YOU'VE GOT RHYTHM

Everyone has a twenty-four-hour internal clock, also called a biological clock, that is regulated by the brain's master clock in the hypothalamus of the brain. This area of the hypothalamus is called the suprachiasmatic nucleus, or SCN. Everyone has their own individualized circadian rhythm or natural sleep/wake cycles. These help to regulate numerous important biological activities such as waking up, sleeping, the release of certain hormones (including melatonin and cortisol), blood pressure, body temperature, blood sugar levels, digestive secretions, and so on.

Our brains are actually programmed for activity during the daylight and are programmed to sleep when it gets dark, based upon our circadian rhythms. Before electricity was developed, almost everyone went to bed when it was dark and awakened whenever it was light outside. Now, however, with the help of bright lights, TVs, computer screens, and more, many have confused their brains into thinking it is daytime when in reality it is the middle of the night. Also, nightclubs, late-night shopping and dining, late-night movies, the Internet, shift work, and artificial lighting have disrupted many people's circadian rhythms or natural sleep/wake cycles. Many have developed insomnia as a result of this.

One's biological clock responds to several external cues, which help to keep it set on a twenty-four-hour schedule. These cues are called *zeitgebers* and include light and melatonin. However, light is the most significant cue.

In order for you to perform at your best, your circadian rhythms or natural sleep/wake cycles need to be synchronized with your work and lifestyle. In the United States, the majority of Americans go to work at 8:00 or 9:00 a.m. and then work until 5:00 or 6:00 p.m. In order to work those hours and get eight hours of sleep at night, most people should go to bed at 10:00 or 11:00 p.m. and wake up at 6:00 or 7:00 a.m. Now, if you have a one- to two-hour commute to work, you will need to go to bed even earlier and wake up earlier.

However, people whose internal biological clock is out of sync typically cannot go to sleep when they need to go to sleep and suffer the consequences as a result. Let's look at a few ways that can happen.

Night owls

Night owls are individuals with delayed sleep phase syndrome (DSPS). They generally stay up late at night and usually do not fall asleep until 2:00 or 3:00 a.m.—or sometimes even later. They then enjoy sleeping until late morning or early afternoon. This is very common with students in high school and college.

The problem for night owls is that most jobs require you to be at work at 8:00 or 9:00 a.m. unless you are lucky enough to find a good job that starts around 2:00 or 3:00 in the afternoon. Good luck with that. Otherwise, you need to adjust your circadian rhythm accordingly. Many musicians and artists have delayed sleep phase syndrome and do not even realize it.

Treatment for delayed sleep phase syndrome for night owls includes chronotherapy, light therapy, and melatonin. Chronotherapy simply delays sleep in two- or three-hour increments daily until the patient's sleeping and waking patterns are normalized. It is fairly difficult to do, and I rarely use it. The patient must closely adhere to this new schedule. For example, with a patient who typically falls asleep at 3:00 a.m. but desires to fall asleep at 11:00 p.m., we would first move his bedtime up to 6:00 a.m. on Friday night, then to 9:00 a.m. on Saturday morning, 12 noon on Sunday, 3:00 p.m. on Monday, 6:00 p.m. on Tuesday, 9:00 p.m. on Wednesday, and finally 11:00 p.m. on Thursday.

Now, in an order to do this, I may also need to give a temporary sleeping pill, such as Ambien or Rozerem. Rozerem helps to shift the circadian rhythms. Also, a supplement may be needed in order to help the patient fall asleep. One also needs to practice sleep hygiene, relaxation techniques, and stress-reduction techniques.

Light therapy, which will be discussed with other therapies in chapter 5, can also treat delayed sleep phase syndrome. Patients with DSPS may also improve with melatonin a few hours before bedtime as the lights are dimmed. I usually recommend 3–6 mg of melatonin dissolved in the mouth.

Early birds

Early birds are patients who have advanced sleep phase syndrome (ASPS) and are the exact opposite of patients with delayed sleep phase syndrome. These individuals usually start getting sleepy around 7:00 or 8:00 p.m. and then awaken between 3:00 and 5:00 a.m. They usually have no trouble falling asleep, have normal sleep architecture, and are not sleepy during the day. However, they usually think they have insomnia because they awaken typically between 3:00 and 5:00 a.m. and simply cannot fall back to sleep. They may lead very boring social lives since they are usually asleep by 8:00 p.m.

This disorder is also treated with light therapy and melatonin. However, early birds do not respond well to chronotherapy. These individuals typically benefit from wearing a light visor or sitting in a light box between 7:00 and 9:00 p.m., which delays their circadian rhythm. Their bedroom must be totally dark; I recommend blackout curtains and covering every little light with black electrical tape. I may treat patients with ASPS with 1 mg of melatonin in the morning to delay the circadian rhythm and a larger dose of 3–6 mg of melatonin at bedtime. It should be taken around 9:00 or 10:00 p.m.

Jet lag

The main symptom of jet lag is severe fatigue. Typically people flying north and south do not experience jet lag since they do not cross any time zones. Individuals traveling east usually experience the worst jet lags since they lose an hour for every time zone they cross.

Typically the brain can adjust its biological clock by an hour or two each day; however, three or more hours is a different story. When you fly from Atlanta to London, you cross five time zones, and even though the local time in London is 9:00 a.m., your body's internal clock still thinks it is 4:00 a.m. Your brain is getting conflicting messages as the sunlight tells your brain to wake up but your internal clock and lack of sleep are telling you to sleep.

Jet lag affects everyone, but there are ways you can minimize these effects. First, start two or three days before a trip when you are crossing three or four time zones by adjusting your watch and clock to the new time zone. Then try to go to bed at the time you normally go to bed, but do so on the new time zone schedule that your watch is now set to. You may want to start the process a few days earlier if you have to cross four or more time zones. I also strongly recommend 3–6 mg of melatonin that is dissolved in the mouth at bedtime and that you maintain good sleep hygiene.

Shift work

Unfortunately most workers doing shift work live in constant disruption of their circadian rhythm. Long-term shift work increases the risk of heart disease. One study found a modest increased risk of breast cancer in long-term employees who work night shift when compared to those who did not.[2]

These individuals need to practice good sleep hygiene and avoid morning sunlight by trying to get home and in bed as soon as possible, preferably before sunrise. Try to minimize exposure to sunlight by wearing dark sunglasses on your drive home that cover the sides and tops of your eyes, preventing sunlight shining in. Make your bedroom as dark as possible with blackout curtains, and soundproof your bedroom to keep daytime noise out. Turn off the phone in your bedroom. Also, it is good to take a twenty-minute power nap once a day if you become fatigued. I also recommend taking 3–6 mg of melatonin dissolved in the mouth at bedtime.

Artificial light pollution

The sky glow of Los Angeles is visible from an airplane approximately two hundred miles away; this is also true of many other cities.[3] Sky glow is simply one form of light pollution. The International Agency for Research on Cancer has classified light at night as a group IIA carcinogen (a probable carcinogen).[4]

Light at night inhibits the nighttime increase of melatonin, which is the hormone that also has oncostatic properties (tumor-prevention properties).

Artificial light also disrupts our circadian rhythm. Whenever light shines on your eyes or even your skin, it stimulates the release of cortisol—the stress hormone that causes your brain to think it is morning. Many people have numerous little lights in their bedroom from their alarm clock, phone, TV components, alarm system, and so on. These artificial lights may be keeping you from a good night's sleep.

The worst type of artificial light at night is green, blue, and white lights. Candlelight, orange, or red light is not nearly as harmful, so when purchasing an alarm clock, do not choose one with a green or blue light, but rather purchase one with a red light. Also, it is important to cover the alarm clock with a hand towel in order to prevent any light from shining on your eyes or even your skin.

There is epidemiological evidence that shows that the incidence of cancer increases in people living in environments where light pollution is high. In animal studies, destruction of the biological clock actually accelerates experimental cancer growth.[5] It is important for us to realize that artificial light is a probable carcinogen. We should then cover all artificial light in our bedrooms and make sure that we have blackout curtains in order to prevent artificial light from streetlights and sky glows from affecting our sleep.

MAKE IT COUNT

As a nation we have become too dependent upon energy drinks and medications to keep us awake longer. We need to realize that when we cheat the body from getting the sleep it needs, we may eventually suffer the consequences healthwise.

We've looked at what can rob you of a good night's sleep. We've also learned that getting the right amount of sleep is vital to optimal performance on a daily basis. Now let's go look at your ideal night of sleep and sleep preparation, which makes all the difference in giving you a good night's rest.

Building Blocks to a Better Night's Sleep

- The length of time you need to sleep varies depending on your age and stage in life.

- You start playing with fire when you don't honor your circadian rhythm—the natural clock inside your body that follows the earth's natural cycles.

- You need at least three to four cycles of sleep a night. Each cycle includes five stages, broken into two parts. The third and fourth stage are the most important and deepest levels of sleep, and the fifth stage is where dreams happen.

Chapter 3

WHAT'S ROBBING YOU OF A GOOD NIGHT'S SLEEP?

ONE TIME I developed a shoulder injury while lifting weights. During the day the pain was annoying, but I could ignore it. At night the pain became major because every time I tried to sleep, I eventually rolled over on that shoulder and woke up. That went on for months, and I became an unwilling insomniac until the shoulder healed. I felt like a walking zombie!

Many of you know exactly how I felt. Everybody wants to sleep well, but many of us can't for reasons that range from troubling life situations to physical problems to poor eating habits. You may even have a serious sleeping disorder, and we will address the various sleeping disorders that need particular care in a later chapter. Suffice it to say that if you have difficulty sleeping, you are not alone. This chapter will identify more common sleep ailments and help you move toward getting the quality of sleep you need regularly.

COMMON SLEEP THIEVES

First, let's talk about the most common deterrents to a good night's sleep.

Stress and anxiety. By far the biggest cause of insomnia is stress. People lie awake trying to work out their life's problems, mourning the past, and worrying about the future.

Painful physical conditions. Arthritis, chronic back pain, tension headaches, degenerative disk disease, bursitis, tendonitis, and virtually any other painful condition can rob an otherwise healthy person of sleep.

Caffeine. Many people doom their sleep by consuming caffeine in coffee, soft drinks, chocolate, and over-the-counter headache medicines like Excedrin. Caffeine increases the stress hormones adrenaline and cortisol. Also, caffeine can remain in the body for up to twenty hours. More than 80 percent of all Americans consume caffeine regularly, and the average American drinks about three cups of coffee a day. For some people, that's a recipe for sleepless nights.

Cigarettes and alcohol. Nicotine and alcohol can interfere with sleep. Some people think alcohol helps you to fall asleep, but in fact alcohol can disrupt the stages of sleep, causing you to sleep lighter and to awaken feeling less refreshed. Nicotine from cigarette smoking is a stimulant that causes adrenaline to be released, which often causes insomnia.

Medications. Decongestants, appetite suppressants, asthma medications (such as theophylline), prednisone, thyroid medications, hormone replacement, some pain relievers, some blood pressure medications, and certain antidepressants may all cause insomnia.

Food insomnia. Many people eat too much sugar and highly processed foods before bed, keeping their nightly date with a bowl of ice cream, piece of cake, or bag of popcorn. These carbohydrates stimulate excessive insulin release from the pancreas. The result is a "sugar high" of energy. But later, usually in the middle of the night, your blood sugar hits a "low," which triggers the adrenal glands to produce more adrenaline and cortisol. Suddenly you are awake and feel hungry again.

Low-carb diets. These diets can also create a low-blood-sugar reaction, causing you to awaken in the middle of the night. Even if you fill up your stomach with healthy foods at bedtime, it may affect the quality of your sleep. When you eat too much protein or eat too late, you generally will need more sleep. This is especially true when you eat too much meat. That's the reason why animals, like lions and tigers, usually require up to twenty hours a day of sleep—their bodies are having to digest and assimilate all the protein in their bellies.

Exercise. People who exercise within three hours of going to sleep raise their levels of stress hormones, which may interfere with sleep.

A bad mattress or pillow. Is there anything more frustrating than a mattress that is too saggy or too hard, or an overstuffed pillow?

A snoring spouse. My neighbor came to me one day and said, "Please give my husband something to stop his snoring! I can't even sleep in the same bed anymore. He snores so loud that our kids in the other bedrooms wake up scared in the middle of the night." Many people feel that desperate. A snoring spouse wrecks many people's sleep. I'll share my remedies for snoring in a later section.

Newborn babies. As welcome as they are, babies can ruin sleep patterns. Breast-feeding mothers know how an active nighttime routine can make their brains and bodies feel like jelly.

Hot flashes or menstrual cramps. Women over fifty often

know the aggravation of being kept awake by hot flashes or night sweats. Other women have such severe cramping that they become insomniacs every month when their period arrives.

Enlarged prostate. Some men over fifty find themselves on a there-and-back-again loop to the bathroom when they should be fast asleep.

Environment. Noisy neighbors and their dogs, the room too hot or too cold, bright lights shining through your bedroom window, or trucks, planes, trains, or motorcycles passing by can all disrupt sleep patterns.

Each of these sleep thieves is responsible for countless hours of lost sleep, lost productivity, lost creativity, and lost mental health.

CONSUMPTION CULPRITS

Let's take a closer look at some of these sleep thieves—in particular, those having to do with what we choose to ingest as food or drink. As you will see, our consumption habits can greatly impact the quality of our sleep.

Caffeine

I am not against drinking one or even two cups of organic coffee in the morning, because of the numerous health benefits of coffee. However, caffeine increases alertness and stimulates the central nervous system. And unfortunately many Americans are drinking coffee or some other caffeinated beverage in the late afternoon or evening, and that is affecting their sleep.

It takes about six hours to metabolize half the caffeine in a small cup of coffee.[1] So if you drink your coffee in the late afternoon or evening, the caffeine will probably stimulate your nervous system and keep you alert during the night, thus prohibiting you from entering the deeper stages of sleep. The more deep sleep you attain usually enables you to awaken more refreshed. If you are suffering from insomnia, limit your coffee intake to one to two cups a day in 8-ounce cups, not 16-ounce size, or approximately 150–300 mg of caffeine a day.

If you have any liver impairment caused by medications such as statin drugs or history of a fatty liver, cut that amount of caffeine in half. If you still have problems with insomnia, keep cutting back your caffeine intake until you have either weaned off coffee or you are sleeping well.

Beware that over-the-counter medications can be packed with caffeine as well. For example, one Excedrin contains 65 mg of caffeine. Cold medications also commonly contain caffeine. So watch your intake of those products before bedtime.

Chocolate can also keep you up at night due to its caffeine component. Chocolate ice cream, chocolate cake, chocolate candy bars, chocolate milk—all of these contain caffeine and theobromine, which are both stimulants. Chocolate also contains tyramine and phenylethylamine, both of which increase alertness and can contribute to insomnia.

Sugar and carbs

Caffeine is not the only dietary enemy of sleep. Sugar can be just as bad for your ability to rest. A poor diet of too many simple sugars and processed carbohydrates can also lead to insomnia. We in America eat far too much sugar, and when we eat sugar before going to bed, sleeplessness can be the result.

Americans are now consuming more fat-free foods, which

usually means they are over-consuming highly processed carbohydrates and sugars. Foods high in processed carbohydrates and sugars stimulate insulin release from the pancreas. Insulin in turn triggers the body to store more fat. Insulin may also cause low blood sugar. Low blood sugar then triggers the adrenals to produce more adrenaline and cortisol, which may cause you to be awakened in the middle of the night.

Eating sugar and processed carbohydrates before bedtime often leads to low blood sugar in the middle of the night. This can also happen if you go to bed hungry. You can prevent this dip in blood sugar that wakes you out of sleep by eating a light, well-balanced, high-fiber snack at bedtime. Eating a light evening snack that is correctly balanced with proteins, carbohydrates, fiber, and fats will stabilize blood sugar levels and improve sleep.

You may use whey protein, rice protein, or a vegetarian protein other than soy (such as Life's Basics). These are protein powders that may be mixed with water, coconut milk, skim milk, or plain low-fat kefir. Or you may get plain protein powder such as whey, vegetarian (such as Life's Basics), or rice and make a smoothie with frozen fruit and ice mixed with water, coconut milk, skim milk, or plain low-fat kefir.

Late-night eating and drinking

When it comes to what keeps you up at night, it's not just what you consume but also when you consume it. Eating a large meal close to bedtime can cause insomnia. Our digestive tract is not designed to digest in a prone or supine (lying) position and works best when we are up and moving around. Our stomach and pancreas are also not designed to be undergoing major digestion of food while we are sleeping. This is another reason we see so much heartburn, indigestion, and acid reflux in America, which also contribute to our insomnia.

Foods containing both tyrosine and tyramine cause insomnia because they are converted in the body to norepinephrine, which is an excitatory neurotransmitter that stimulates us and may keep us awake. Foods high in tyrosine include milk, cheese, yogurt, cottage cheese, soy, peanuts, bananas, turkey, and lima beans. Foods that are high in tyramine include red wine; yogurt; sour cream; aged cheeses; pickled meats; many fish; fermented foods such as soy sauce, sauerkraut, and pickles; figs; raisins; dates; fresh baked breads; and processed meats such as bologna and salami.

Also, consuming too many fatty foods close to bedtime will delay digestion and can cause insomnia. Fats take much longer to digest compared with carbohydrates or proteins.

Let's not forget one more culprit: alcohol. Many individuals drink one or two glasses of wine at night since it helps them unwind and fall asleep. Yes, as I mentioned previously, alcohol does help you fall asleep; however, you are more likely to awaken later in the night. Alcohol intake reduces the time spent in stages three and four and REM sleep, which are the most restorative stages of sleep.

What's more, alcohol can worsen snoring. So, alcohol is actually a double-edged sword when it comes to sleep. Also, a major problem with many of my patients is overconsumption of fluids in the evening. As a result, they are up two to three times a night urinating. After 7:00 p.m. simply cut back on your fluid intake.

Dr. Colbert Approved Bedtime Snacks

- A piece of fruit, like a small apple, grapefruit, 4 ounces of berries or kiwi with a small handful of nuts (walnuts, almonds, or pecans)
- One serving of low-fat, whole-grain crackers or one piece of whole-grain bread with about a teaspoon of organic peanut butter or two ounces of turkey
- One-half cup organic skim milk or low-fat cottage cheese or low-fat, no-sugar yogurt (if not sensitive to dairy) with fruit added
- A small bowl of whole-grain cereal (about ½ cup) with organic skim milk

THE CASE OF THE SNORING SPOUSE

Does your partner happily saw logs all night while you watch the ceiling? If your spouse snores, it could be sign of sleep apnea (which we will discuss in a later chapter on sleep disorders). But know that even though all patients with sleep apnea snore, all snorers do not have sleep apnea. Have your partner undergo a medical evaluation if he or she seems to stop breathing for short periods of time.

Snoring that is not related to sleep apnea does not pose any health risks and does not cause daytime drowsiness for the snorer. However, it does cause problems for the snorer's spouse. Snoring is also fairly difficult to cure.

Snoring is one of the most common sleep problems in the United States, affecting about 42 percent of men and 31 percent of women.[2] Those who snore often have anatomical differences, such as an obstructed nasal passage, a deviated nasal septum, or an elongation of the uvula (the tissue that hangs down the back of the throat). The snoring may also be due to sagging of the soft palate. Enlarged tonsils or adenoids can cause snoring too, as well as poor muscle tone in the tissues of the soft palate, throat, and tongue.

Gaining weight usually increases snoring simply because the body eventually deposits the extra fat in the lining of the throat, causing the breathing passages to narrow more and more. Also, the uvula actually elongates as we age and gain weight.

If your spouse is an overweight snorer, losing weight and exercising is the best advice for him or her—a weight loss of just 10 to 15 pounds can make a big difference!

Changing sleeping positions can also help. Try sewing a pocket into the back of a T-shirt and placing a tennis ball or a plastic ball in it to keep your happy snorer from sleeping on his back.

If your spouse's weight or sleeping position is not the issue, there may be other common triggers of snoring. Is it nasal congestion, a deviated nasal septum, enlarged tonsils or adenoids, or decreased muscle tone in the throat with a sagging uvula or soft palate? Is it alcohol or medication?

For nasal congestion I generally recommend a homeopathic herbal over-the-counter decongestant, which generally helps. Breathe Right strips, a decongestant, or a nasal steroid such as Flonase or Nasonex will help to open the nasal passages and may prevent snoring. Your spouse may also benefit from using a humidifier or snoring sprays, which simply lubricate the back of the throat with some type of oil, such as olive oil, almond oil, or grape seed oil. These oils help prevent the soft tissues from sticking together.

Other things to do include avoiding alcohol, muscle relaxants, tranquilizers, and sleep medications since they tend to relax the muscles of the throat, which can worsen snoring. Cigarette smoke can also cause the tissues of the throat to swell and thus encourage snoring.

Many snorers have a sagging uvula or soft palate. Dental devices are reported to help many snorers. There are more than fifty different variations available. These are usually either a mandibular-advancing device, which advances the lower jaw, or a tongue-retaining device that holds the tongue forward. These devices are usually purchased from dentists who are specifically trained in treating patients who snore. Or you can also purchase a snore alarm at specialty stores. A snore alarm is simply a wristwatch that vibrates as soon a person begins to snore.

When severe snoring persists even after trying the above techniques, especially in the case of a deviated septum or enlarged adenoids, you might consider surgery. However, for a sagging soft palate or uvula, I would first recommend trying somnoplasty. Somnoplasty uses radiofrequency ablation to shrink the soft tissues of the soft palate. It is performed as an outpatient procedure under local anesthesia. A tiny probe sends out radio waves that shrink the tissues. There is minimal pain with or after the procedure and minimal post-op complications. It may need to be repeated to achieve the best results.

If you're the nonsnoring spouse, you might also try a background noise machine (which can be purchased at Brookstone). The sound of a waterfall, raindrops, or white noise can usually drown out a snoring spouse. You might also get some soft earplugs until your snoring partner has been treated, or, if none of the above measures help, consider sleeping in another bedroom.

Control the Snore

There is a fairly new procedure using radio frequency waves to help shrink the uvula and soft palate. The US Food and Drug Administration has approved a treatment for snoring that uses radio waves to shrink tissue in air passages and eliminate snoring. The procedure is called radiofrequency volumetric tissue reduction of the palate. The radiofrequency treatment involves piercing the tongue, throat, or soft palate with a special needle (electrode) connected to a radio frequency generator. The inner tissue is then heated to 8 to 76 degrees in a procedure that takes approximately half an hour. The inner tissues shrink, but the outer tissues, which may contain such things as taste buds, are left intact. Several treatments may be required.[3]

Getting Ready for Nighttime

We've looked at what can rob you of a good night's sleep. We have also learned that getting the right amount of sleep is vital to optimal performance on a daily basis. Now let's go through your ideal night of sleep and sleep preparation together, which should start earlier than you might think.

Start in the afternoon

Preparing for sleep at night begins during the daytime. Engage in some sort of aerobic exercise, such as brisk walking in the afternoon or early evening. Daily exercise is one of the best ways to improve the quality of your sleep because it helps you fall asleep faster and sleep longer. People who exercise spend a greater amount of time in stage three and four sleep, the most restorative and repairing stages of sleep.

But don't go overboard and rev up your body with exercise within three hours of bedtime. It heats up your body and raises the stress hormones. Not long ago I took a sauna too close to bedtime and got so hot that I couldn't sleep well. What a mistake!

Eat a modest, healthy dinner four hours before bedtime. You may eat a light evening snack before bed—even better is a snack that is correctly balanced with proteins, carbohydrates, and fats. This snack will help stabilize blood sugar through the nighttime hours. Some people can handle caffeine; others can't. If you fall in the latter category, then quit drinking or eating caffeinated products by noon.

As the sun goes down, your body will relax naturally. You are designed hormonally to stay in sync with the cycles of nature. When the light fades, the hormone melatonin is released into your bloodstream, making you sleepy. The amount of melatonin your body produces is affected by the amount of light going into your eyes. That's why you are more alert and energetic on sunny days and more lethargic on cloudy days. It's also why some people can work all night staring at a computer or television screen, because they are feeding light into their eyes.

Follow your body's signal and turn down the lights as the sun goes down. Light messes up our hormonal response at night. I tell patients to buy dimmer switches so they can bring the lights down. If you have the money and time, get a massage in the late afternoon. If you don't have the money, but you do have a spouse, exchange massages with him or her. If you don't have a spouse, buy a handheld massager at a store like Brookstone or The Sharper Image.

Slow your input

Don't watch an action-packed movie or even the late local news program, which tends to play up violent news stories. Watch something calming, play your favorite soothing music, or perhaps watch a funny TV show or movie since laughter helps to relax you. Take a warm shower or bath, adding soothing salts or lavender oil. (Epsom salt has magnesium, which relaxes the body.) Get all your senses involved. Dim the lights, listen to music, and relax.

In the fall season I break all these rules once a week because of a sports tradition I can't let go of: Monday Night Football. I unrepentantly watch the game and get all worked up, and my sleep takes a hit that night, especially when the game goes into overtime. To me it's worth it, and I usually recover fine because I sleep properly the other six nights of the week. But as a doctor, I don't recommend getting hooked on habits that interfere with sleep.

Corral your thoughts

As the evening goes on and your mind wanders over the events of the day, don't let anxiety derail you from your goal. Switch from the "worry" channel to the "appreciation and praise" channel. Make a list of things for which you are thankful, and then dwell on those instead.

One woman I treated had gone through a divorce and developed a serious sleep problem. She would wake up at 2:00 or 3:00 a.m., and she would lie in bed and rehash the whole failed relationship—every detail, what she did, what he did, what she should and shouldn't have done. She could not figure out why he left her. She wanted a sense of peace, but her mind would not let her sleep.

Mary and I had to teach this divorced woman how to change her thoughts. I gave her a prescription—to read the Bible. I had her write out promises from the Bible and keep them by her bedside. Before she turned in, she read them and laid her problems in God's hands. I had her memorize verses from the Bible, so when she woke up she wouldn't have to turn on the light—which would stimulate her mind—but could quote the Bible from memory.

Instead of focusing on her problems, I had her corral her thoughts and focus on God's Word, which is the answer. I had her meditate on 1 Corinthians 13:4–8, which is the love walk. We'll talk more about handling stress and anxiety, as well as tuning our thoughts toward gratitude and God's promises in later chapters.

Plan your bedtime

In my opinion, sleep before midnight is better than sleep after midnight. If you can't bear the idea of going to sleep that "early," remember that your very health is at stake. Ninety to 95 percent of your sixty to one hundred trillion cells are replaced each year, and much of that occurs during sleep that comes early in the night. Not only that, but while you sleep, your body rejuvenates itself.[4] Sleep and water are the two best antiaging secrets I have found. If you value your looks and your life span, getting to bed at 10:00 p.m. won't be difficult. For many patients with chronic disease, the most important recommendation I can give them is to be in bed by 9:00 p.m. and to sleep at least eight hours. God designed us to fall asleep when it is dark and to wake up when the sun rises.

Create a sleep haven

When you walk into your bedroom, it should look like an inviting place of rest—not a storage unit. Some women use their bedrooms for all their projects, surrounding the bed with stacks of magazines, sewing supplies, half-finished blankets, books, and family photos waiting to be put in albums. Then they cover the bed with the laundry they did earlier and the outfits they considered wearing that morning. This scene causes clutter stress. If you wonder why you and your husband start arguing as soon as you walk into your bedroom, maybe it's the clutter that assaults your eyes.

Men are just as bad. Some men turn their bedroom into their home office or video game room. Nestled conspicuously in the corner is a computer desk, a whirring CPU, stacks of receipts, and important papers. Small wonder that when you walk into the room, your mind is conflicted: "Is this where I sleep, work, or play?" All that stress comes on you at precisely the wrong time.

Make your bedroom a haven for sleep and unwinding. Have some rules: No eating, no computers, no harsh clock lights, and no televisions, if you can stand it. No studying, no sewing projects, no stacks of laundry waiting to be folded and put away, no piles of junk you shoved in there when the neighbor came over to visit. Your bedroom should say one thing: sleep!

Make your bed and lie in it

Your bed should be more comfortable than your couch. After all, you don't spend eight hours a day on the couch, but you do on your mattress. One of the best investments you can make for your health is a mattress you thoroughly enjoy and look forward to lying on. The same goes for your pillow. Treat these like a secret source of happiness, which you anticipate every day.

A mattress that is too firm does not adequately allow for the right alignment of the spine. A mattress that is too soft will allow the spine to sag and may cause a backache. When you shop for a mattress, don't just lie on your back; also lie on your side and your stomach. Slide your hand, palm down, between the mattress and the small of your back as you try lying on your back. If you are able to get your entire hand through the small of your back, the mattress is too hard. If while lying flat on the bed the base of the spine is lower than your heels, the mattress is too soft.

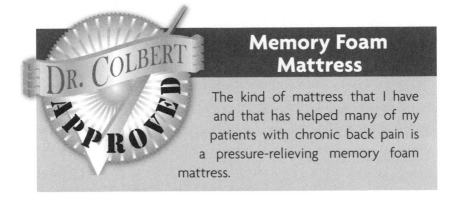

DR. COLBERT APPROVED

Memory Foam Mattress

The kind of mattress that I have and that has helped many of my patients with chronic back pain is a pressure-relieving memory foam mattress.

If your pillow is too hard, too soft, too large, or too small, your quality of sleep may suffer. Select the right pillow for you. A pillow should be soft enough to conform to the contours of your head and neck, but also thick enough to support the head and neck in a neutral position.

The room should be as dark as you can reasonably make it. Don't have nightlights, and don't let streetlights shine through the window. Line the drapes, or pull down a dark shade if you need to. If you are routinely awakened by sirens, car alarms, horns, roaring motorcycles, coyotes, airplanes—whatever noisemakers roam freely in your area during the night—invest in double-pane windows or maybe a good set of soft earplugs. Or buy a sound generator that makes waterfall or raindrop sounds. If you tend to get unwanted calls, get the call block feature from your phone service provider or take the phone off the hook.

I noted earlier that some people wake up because their blood sugar level drops. Eat some of the snacks mentioned previously. That will balance out your blood sugar level for the evening.

The room should be at a comfortable temperature, usually around 70 to 75 degrees Fahrenheit. Some people like to open the windows, especially if they live in the mountains or at the beach, and let the cool air come in while they huddle under warm blankets. Others like a warmer ambient temperature. Some prefer the feeling of a ceiling fan, which improves airflow. Figure out what works best for you and your spouse, and stick with it.

TWENTY-FIVE SLEEP HABITS THAT HELP

As you continue to develop good health habits to improve the quality of your sleep, consider adopting good sleep hygiene. Sleep hygiene simply refers to the practices that promote continuous and effective sleep. Another way to look at it is this: sleep hygiene is simply establishing healthy sleep habits. There are twenty-five good sleep hygiene habits that will enable most people to fall asleep and stay asleep.[5]

1. The most important sleep hygiene tip is to establish a regular bedtime as well as a regular time of waking up in the morning. Make this a habit, and stick to the schedule on weekends and even during vacations. Do not be haphazard about it, but based on your work schedule, set aside eight hours for sleep and a time to be in bed. For myself, I choose to be in bed between 10:00 and 10:30 p.m.

2. Use your bed only for sleep and sexual relations. Do not use your bed for reading, watching TV, snacking, working, or worrying.

3. Avoid naps after 3:00 p.m. When they are taken earlier in the day, make sure they are not longer than twenty to thirty minutes.

4. Exercise before dinner. Exercising too close to bedtime disrupts sleep.

5. Avoid caffeine in the late afternoon and evening.

6. Avoid excessive fluids in the late evening and especially before bedtime.

7. Eat normal portion sizes of a well-balanced meal at dinnertime approximately three to four hours before bedtime as well as a light bedtime snack. Do not go to bed hungry, and do not eat a large meal prior to bedtime.

8. Take a warm bath one to two hours before bedtime, and consider adding lavender oil if desired in order to help you relax.

9. Keep the bedroom cool and well ventilated.

10. Purchase a comfortable mattress, pillow, and linens. (Check out a 3-inch Tempur-Pedic pad to put on top of your mattress.) Remember, you spend roughly one-third of your life in bed; therefore, your bed should be your most important piece of furniture.

11. Thirty minutes before going to bed, start to wind down by listening to soothing music,

reading the Bible or another good book, having a massage, or being intimate with your spouse.

12. Put dimmer switches on your lights, and dim them a few hours prior to bedtime.

13. After you lie down to go to sleep, if you are not asleep in twenty minutes, simply get up, go into another room, and read and relax in dim light until you feel sleepy. Then return to bed.

14. If your spouse awakens you with snoring or unusual movements, simply move to the guest bedroom.

15. Try to wake up at the same time each day.

16. Try exchanging foot, neck and shoulder, back, or scalp massages with your spouse, and purchase an inexpensive handheld massager from Brookstone.

17. Relax your mind and body before bedtime by gentle stretching, relaxation exercises, or using an aromatherapy candle or oil.

18. Clean clutter out of the bedroom, and remove computers, fax machines, paperwork, and anything that reminds you of work.

19. Make sure your bedroom is completely dark. Remove all nightlights, and cover your alarm clock and phone light with a hand towel. Put

black electrical tape or sticky notepads over tiny lights on your alarm system, TV, DVD, satellite, stereo, or any other lights that are visible. Consider purchasing blackout curtains.

20. Block out noise by using earplugs, double-paning your windows, or using heavy drapes. I personally use a sound generator I purchased from Brookstone that plays white noise. Or you can simply use a fan.

21. Try a lullaby CD or a CD that has sounds of nature.

22. Keep pets out of your bedroom. Pets may snore, pounce on you, growl, howl, bark, or whine. They can also trigger allergies in many patients.

23. Avoid watching heart-pounding movies, ball games, or late-night news. Instead watch something funny or lighthearted before bedtime, but it's best not to watch TV in the bedroom.

24. When lying in bed, you and your spouse may try telling or reading funny jokes to one another. Couples who laugh together and pray together generally stay together.

25. Meditate on Scripture, and do not let your mind worry or wander. I meditate on the Lord's Prayer in Matthew 6:9–13. I also meditate on Psalm 91, 1 Corinthians 13:4–8, and Ephesians

6:10–18. You need to memorize these scriptures and meditate on them over and over.

KEEP A SLEEP DIARY

Making sure your body benefits from all the stages of sleep can be a challenge, as we have seen earlier with so many Americans getting so little sleep each night, but you do not have to be one of the statistics. I recommend keeping a sleep diary because it will enable you to make some key observations in order to determine your true sleep problem. Complete your sleep diary each morning upon waking. If you are taking sleep aids, please refrain from taking them while you are keeping this sleep diary so that you can know the pure details of your sleep issue. Please be sure to include the following information in your diary:

1. The time you went to bed and the time you woke up

2. How long it took you to fall asleep

3. The times you woke up during the night and how long it took you to fall back asleep

4. How much caffeine you consumed during the day and the time that you consumed it

5. Anything you ate as a meal or snack in the evening and the time you ate it

6. Any naps you took

7. Any medications you took

8. Rating of the quality of your sleep in terms of restful with no awakenings, to few awakenings, frequent awakenings, awakened but fell back to sleep, and finally, awakened and stayed awake

9. Your level of mental alertness when you woke up in the morning (Were you groggy or refreshed?)

10. Any physical, emotional, or environmental factors that disturbed your sleep (a snoring spouse, a hot room, television noise, traffic noise, a storm, attending to the needs of a child, stress, recurrent preoccupations, worrisome thoughts, heartburn, coughing, illness, and so on)

It is best to keep a sleep diary for two to four weeks continuously; date each day. When you awaken in the morning (not in the middle of the night), simply write down your observations before you get out of bed.

By now you've discovered that many of your daily choices can impact your ability to walk in the wonderful blessing of refreshing, rejuvenating sleep. Enjoying rest is a powerful gift from God. Therefore, always look to Him for blessed rest, for He promises to give you sleep. The Bible says, "It is vain for you to rise up early, to sit up late, to eat the bread of sorrows; for so He gives His beloved sleep" (Ps. 127:2).

Building Blocks to a Better Night's Sleep

- Sleep thieves hide in unsuspecting places—in food, in artificial light, in medication, in exercise, in your bedroom environment, and even sometimes in your sleep partner. Do all you can to eradicate sleep thieves from your nightly routine.

- Good sleep hygiene is real. Try to incorporate all twenty-five habits into your lifestyle of rest.

- A sleep diary can help you notice patterns and problems. Use it to track your nightly rest.

Chapter 4

SLEEP DISORDERS

I F YOU DRAG through your days feeling tired and spend too many nights staring at the ceiling or wandering around your house, you may be one of millions of Americans who suffer from a sleep disorder. Sleep disorders are at epidemic levels in the United States. An estimated sixty million Americans suffer from insomnia and other sleep disorders. Other reports state that 60 percent of American adults suffer from insomnia at least a few times each week. As a result, more than half of the population will experience daytime drowsiness.[1]

The key to discovering a sleep disorder is how you feel when you wake up and how alert you feel throughout the day. If you do not wake up feeling refreshed and you get sleepy during the day, you may be experiencing a disorder that is robbing your body and mind of much-needed rest each night.

WHICH KIND IS YOURS?

Sleep disorders fall into two main categories:

1. Dyssomnias—characterized by problems
   with either falling asleep or staying asleep,

followed by excessive drowsiness during the day. Examples of dyssomnias include insomnia, sleep apnea, narcolepsy, restless legs syndrome, periodic limb movements, and advanced and delayed sleep phase syndrome.

2. Parasomnias—abnormalities in behavior that occur during sleep, such as night terrors (a frightening activity during sleep), nightmares, sleepwalking and/or sleep talking, bruxism (or grinding your teeth), sleep-related eating disorder, and REM sleep behavior disorder

Let's investigate some of these extremely unpleasant sleeping problems.

INSOMNIA

Insomnia is by far the most common sleep disorder. It is characterized by having problems either falling asleep or staying asleep. There are two main forms of insomnia: primary insomnia and secondary insomnia.

Primary insomnia

Primary insomnia is not due to medical, psychiatric, or environmental problems, nor is it due to medications or any other substances. The insomnia is its own disorder, which means the insomnia is the medical condition and not a symptom of some other medical or psychiatric disease.

Usually primary insomnia is a lone disorder that develops over time. Studies have shown that people with chronic insomnia produce higher levels of stress hormones than other people. Since primary insomnia is its own disorder and is usually associated with stress, I strongly recommend that you read my book *Stress Less*. Using behavioral techniques, sleep hygiene techniques, relaxation techniques, and nutritional supplements will generally help to reverse primary insomnia. These methods will be discussed in detail later in this book.

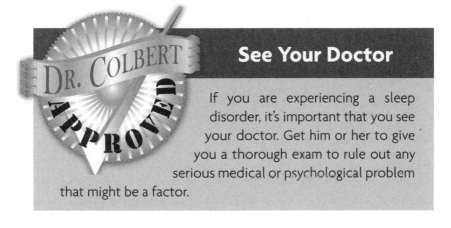

See Your Doctor

If you are experiencing a sleep disorder, it's important that you see your doctor. Get him or her to give you a thorough exam to rule out any serious medical or psychological problem that might be a factor.

Secondary insomnia

The most common type of insomnia, secondary insomnia is a symptom or side effect of some other medical or emotional problem such as anxiety, depression, chronic pain, heart failure, asthma, acid reflux, menopause with hot flashes and night sweats, urological disorders, and so forth. Secondary insomnia can also be due to a side effect of certain medications, especially cold and sinus medications, asthma medications, and more. Secondary insomnia may also be due to caffeine, nicotine, or alcohol.

It is believed that more than eight out of ten people with insomnia suffer from secondary insomnia. Since over 80 percent of patients with insomnia have secondary insomnia, it is critically important to treat the primary problem.[2]

For example, if your insomnia is due to an enlarged prostate and you have to get up multiple times during the night to urinate, simply treating the enlarged prostate will generally correct the insomnia. Also, if your insomnia is due to hot flashes or acid reflux, simply treating the hot flashes or acid reflux will generally get rid of the insomnia. If your insomnia is due to anxiety or depression, then simply treating the anxiety and depression will usually take care of the insomnia.

The good news is that controlling secondary insomnia is fairly easy. Usually this is accomplished by simply treating the primary problem, employing a few behavioral techniques, and following a regimen of sleep hygiene and a few natural supplements.

SLEEP APNEA

Sleep apnea affects over eighteen million Americans, and approximately ten million Americans are not even diagnosed. More than 50 percent of all the patients with sleep apnea are over forty years of age.

Sleep apnea is more common in men than women, with 49 percent of middle-aged men with apnea and only 2–4 percent of middle-aged women with apnea.[3] After menopause women lose the protective effect of estrogen and progesterone, and the risk of developing obstructive sleep apnea increases significantly, nearly to the rate seen in men.

African Americans have a higher risk of sleep apnea than any other ethnic group.

Sleep apnea may eventually lead to hypertension, arrhythmias, congestive heart failure, stroke, coronary artery disease, heart attacks, cardiac arrest, pulmonary hypertension, type 2 diabetes, memory loss, and depression. One study found that one's risk of stroke doubles over a seven-year period if one has sleep apnea.[4]

Sleep apnea is believed to have contributed to the death of football Hall of Famer Reggie White.[5] Sleep apnea is also associated with severe fatigue and daytime sleepiness, memory loss, irritability, accidents, and premature death.

How does one differentiate snoring from the potentially deadly sleep apnea? Well, first of all, the symptoms are usually different with sleep apnea. A patient with sleep apnea usually has severely loud snoring, which is usually interrupted with extended times of silence followed by a gasping, choking, or snorting sound.

People who sleep alone are many times not even aware that they snore or stop breathing, but they usually have specific signs and symptoms of sleep apnea that can still be recognized.

These patients usually have a large neck. Men with sleep apnea usually have a neck circumference greater than 17 inches, and many times much larger than this. Females usually have a neck circumference greater than 16 inches.

They also usually have extreme daytime sleepiness and tend to fall asleep whenever they get quiet for a few minutes, such as at the movies or sitting at one's desk after eating lunch or even during a business meeting. They also commonly feel spacey or like they are in a fog.

Gaining weight also increases a person's risk of developing sleep apnea; conversely, sleep apnea increases their risk of gaining even more weight! This is primarily because people with sleep apnea are usually too tired to do any type of exercise.

People with sleep apnea also usually have problems with

concentration, memory, reaction time, and learning. Their brains have been deprived of oxygen, and they are usually simply exhausted from the lack of quality sleep.

Continued oxygen deprivation places a strain on the heart and lungs and eventually may raise the blood pressure as the vital organs are literally being starved of oxygen. This is why people with sleep apnea have an increased risk of hypertension, heart problems (including heart attacks and cardiac arrest), type 2 diabetes, and even depression.

Family history of sleep apnea typically increases a person's risk of sleep apnea two to four times.

During a sleep apnea episode breathing can stop for about ten seconds to as long as a minute. You then wake up to breathe and typically awaken gasping for air. This cycle of waking up to breathe can occur hundreds of times a night.

There are three kinds of sleep apnea: obstructive sleep apnea, central sleep apnea, and mixed sleep apnea.

Obstructive sleep apnea

Obstructive sleep apnea is the most common type of this very serious disorder, occurring in about 2 to 4 percent of all middle-aged adults.[6] Most people with sleep apnea don't even realize they suffer from it!

In this condition the upper airway becomes completely obstructed for ten seconds or longer. During these episodes blood levels of oxygen decrease and carbon dioxide levels increase.

It's this change in the blood gases that alerts the sleeper's brain that the lungs need to start breathing again. But for this to occur, the brain must awaken the body from sleep. These apneic episodes may occur twenty to hundreds of times a night, awaking the sleeper each time—although he may not realize it. As you can imagine, the result is daytime drowsiness, depression, and learning and memory problems.

It is often found that individuals who have sleep apnea are overweight.[7] In addition, if a man or woman has a large neck, a double chin, and truncal obesity (obesity around the abdominal region), there seems to be an increased correlation with obstructive sleep apnea also. The larger the neck size and the more alcohol that is consumed, the higher the correlation with this sleep disorder.[8]

In order to diagnose sleep apnea, you need to undergo a sleep study at a sleep lab. A sleep study usually measures oxygen saturation, episodes of apnea, body movements, body temperature, pulse, respiration, eye movement, and brain activity. All sleep labs allow sleep in a comfortable environment.

Sleep apnea is usually treated with CPAP (continuous positive airway pressure) or BiPAP (bilevel positive airway pressure). AVAPS (average volume assured pressure support) is a new technology in treating sleep apnea introduced into the United States in 2007. It ensures an adequate depth of breathing and is a special feature to some special BiPAP machines. Also, newer models of CPAP machines are quieter and lighter and have many options and a variety of mask styles.

Years ago some of my patients on CPAP machines would literally jerk their mask off their face in the middle of the night and throw them across the room. Now there are new, very comfortable models that fit the face and nose well. Weight loss and especially decreasing your neck size are often useful in relieving or decreasing the severity of sleep apnea. Somnoplasty may also benefit those with mild sleep apnea.

As you lose weight, be sure that you exercise, which usually helps to decrease your neck size. Additional information on this subject can be found in my books *The Seven Pillars of Health* and *The New Bible Cure for Weight Loss*.

Central sleep apnea

Central sleep apnea occurs when the brain's respiratory centers do not send a message to start breathing. This type of sleep apnea is common in those with congestive heart failure, chronic obstructive pulmonary disease (COPD), as well as neurologic diseases. Therapy is typically aimed at treating the underlying medical problems such as congestive heart failure.

Mixed sleep apnea

Mixed sleep apnea is a combination of obstructive sleep apnea and central sleep apnea, but it is also a result of an obstructed airway.

NARCOLEPSY

Narcolepsy is rare and affects as many as two hundred thousand Americans, and as many as 12 percent have a close relative with the disease.[9] Narcolepsy is a neurological sleep disorder where the brain does not properly regulate the daily cycle of sleep and wakefulness. In other words, the brain is unable to regulate the sleep/wake cycles normally, and the patients suffer from REM sleep abnormality.

Patients with narcolepsy become drowsy during the day and may fall asleep at an inappropriate time, such as during an important business meeting. They also may experience sleep paralysis, cataplexy, hallucinations, and insomnia.

Cataplexy is a sudden loss of muscle function while awake, is usually brief, and occurs in approximately 70 percent of patients with narcolepsy.[10] This may occur with any strong emotion, including anger or laughter. In severe cases the muscles become paralyzed and the person may drop to the floor. About 50 percent of patients with narcolepsy also suffer from sleep paralysis. They are typically unable to move or talk for a few minutes when they are falling asleep or when they are waking up.[11] Also, approximately 50 percent experience hallucinations, which may be frightening sounds, feelings, or images from dreams as they are falling asleep or waking up.[12]

If an individual has severe sleepiness during the day and cataplexy, he or she most likely has narcolepsy. These patients should have a sleep study in order to diagnose narcolepsy. I find that most of these patients also have severe adrenal fatigue. Many patients with narcolepsy will also need a medication such as Provigil, which promotes wakefulness and has few side effects.

Again, a regular bedtime schedule, sleep hygiene, stress reduction techniques, and relaxation techniques may help many with narcolepsy. Support groups are also important for those with narcolepsy. Supplements to help adrenal fatigue are found in my book *Stress Less*.

MOVEMENT DISORDERS

Two movement disorders frequently cause insomnia: restless legs syndrome and periodic limb movement disorder. These movement disorders are actually neurological sleep disorders. Restless legs syndrome usually keeps a person awake, whereas periodic limb movement disorder usually keeps a person's spouse awake. Let's look at each disorder.

Restless legs syndrome (RLS)

Restless legs syndrome affects as many as 12 million Americans.[13] It is a neurological sleep disorder that is characterized by an urge to move the legs, strange feelings in the legs (especially the calves), crawling sensations (like worms crawling on the skin) in the legs, as well as pulling sensations, tingling, and prickling sensations.

These sensations usually start in the evening, but they also may occur in the daytime as a person sits at a desk, watches TV, or even plays. The sensations usually worsen when a person lies down for sleep.

Simply moving your legs or pacing, massaging, or stretching your legs usually relieves the discomfort temporarily; it also helps you cope temporarily. But since these sensations usually occur at night when lying in bed, they can seriously interfere with sleep, causing you to get in and out of bed repeatedly during the night. Over time you will become exhausted and more prone to develop depression.

The cause of RLS is unknown, but it is believed to be a glitch in the neurological pathways through which the brain controls movement and is believed to involve the neurotransmitter dopamine. This disorder does run in families, and a child of a patient with RLS has a 50 percent risk of inheriting it.[14]

Restless legs syndrome is also associated with other medical conditions, including iron-deficiency anemia, diabetes, kidney failure, neuropathy, arthritis, and Parkinson's disease. Also, certain medications can make it worse, including lithium, antihistamines, and antidepressants. Excessive caffeine, nicotine, and stress can also worsen it.

RLS is more common after age fifty.[15] Moderate aerobic exercise such as cycling or walking usually helps to decrease symptoms, whereas excessive exercise may worsen symptoms. Taking a warm bath with 1–4 cups of Epsom salts (hydrated magnesium sulfate) added to your bathwater may also help decrease symptoms.

If you have RLS, your doctor should run blood tests to check for anemia. You should also have your iron, ferritin, and magnesium levels checked. In addition, I recommend that your doctor check for diabetes or kidney problems.

Iron and magnesium supplements may help you with restless legs syndrome, but only take iron supplements if your blood test shows that you are anemic and have low iron levels.

Most men and postmenopausal women should not need iron supplements; if they are anemic, it may be due to a slow GI bleed, colon cancer, ulcer, gastritis, hemorrhoids, or acid reflux. You need to be evaluated by a primary care physician and usually a GI specialist if this is the case.

I also recommend cutting back on caffeine and stopping nicotine as well as alcohol. Stretching exercises, relaxation yoga, massaging the legs, and using heating pads often help to relieve RLS. I always place patients with RLS on a comprehensive multivitamin with a chelated magnesium supplement and a fish oil supplement. This may provide significant relief within a few weeks.

If your restless legs syndrome is very severe and affecting your sleep significantly, talk to your doctor about a medication called Requip, which usually provides significant relief. This medication is very helpful and approved for treating RLS; it is also used to treat Parkinson's disease.

Periodic limb movement disorder (PLMD)

Periodic limb movement disorder is associated with involuntary contractions and movements of the legs and occasionally the arms while one is sleeping. These movements of the legs are typically jerking or kicking movements that last about thirty seconds and may occur hundreds of times a night.

It is different from restless legs syndrome, which occurs when one is awake and the movements are voluntary. PLMD, on the other hand, occurs while one is asleep and the movements are involuntary.

Many patients with PLMD are not even aware that their legs jerk in their sleep. However, their spouse is usually very aware. Usually the spouse is the one being awakened many times during the night and is the one suffering from insomnia, not the offender.

This neurological sleep disorder is also probably related to the neurotransmitter dopamine and is more common in elderly individuals. I treat this disorder similar to RLS and run the same blood tests as RLS. I also put patients with PLMD on a comprehensive multivitamin, chelated magnesium, and fish oil. If their condition is severe, they will also usually benefit from the medication Requip.

PARASOMNIAS

Parasomnias are simply sleep disorders that cause strange behaviors while one is asleep. Let us look at some of the most common parasomnias.

Nightmares

Nightmares occur during REM sleep, or dream sleep. The sleeper is not confused or disoriented and recalls the dream. He or she usually does not have the physical symptoms associated with night terrors either.

Nightmares are frightening dreams that are usually related to a shocking or frightening experience. Certain medications—including narcotics, antidepressants, and sleep aids—may cause nightmares as a side effect. Also, alcohol and drug abuse may be associated with nightmares. Nightmares are common when one is weaning off or stopping benzodiazepines, such as Xanax or Valium, or weaning off alcohol or barbiturates. Even certain foods such as chocolate may cause nightmares. They occur in up to 7 percent of adults and are more common in children.[16]

However, good sleep hygiene and regular bedtimes are very important in overcoming nightmares. Refusing to watch any scary movies or TV shows and even late-night news is also very important. If nightmares do not improve, we generally recommend cognitive-behavioral therapy and/or counseling.

I commonly help patients with nightmares using acupressure techniques in order to remove traumatic triggers.

Night terrors

Night terrors are entirely different from nightmares. In night terrors the sleeper usually has no memory or little memory of the episode. He or she usually awakens disoriented and confused and typically experiences increased pulse, increased blood pressure, sweating, rapid breathing, extreme agitation, and dilated pupils.

The sleeper also usually sits up in bed, terrified, and

screams a terrifying scream. He then may gasp, moan, or thrash on the bed. Sometimes sleepwalking can accompany night terrors.

This disorder is not associated with dreaming, but it occurs during non-REM sleep; the sleeper is simply caught in between sleep and awakening.

Children tend to suffer more from night terrors than adults, with up to 6 percent of children and less than 1 percent of adults experiencing them.[17] Children typically outgrow them.

When a child or adult experiences a night terror, simply talk to him quietly in a comforting voice. Be careful to touch him only when he is calming down, since the touch may be misinterpreted as an attack.

It is also very important to maintain a regular sleep time to avoid sleep deprivation. Read your child a lighthearted bedtime story and not a scary story to help relieve his or her stress and anxiety. Cognitive-behavioral therapy or counseling may also be helpful in some individuals. We also use acupressure techniques that are a combination of applied kinesiology and acupressure that helps relieve fear, anxiety, and stress, as well as other techniques to help identify and remove any traumatic triggers. Also, remove caffeinated beverages from the diet, especially in the late afternoon and evening time.

Sleepwalking

Sleepwalking (somnambulism) is very common in children, with as many as 15 percent of school-age children sleepwalking at least once and approximately 1 percent of adults sleepwalking.[18]

Usually treatment for sleepwalking is not necessary since

most will eventually outgrow it. However, if someone is prone to injure himself through sleepwalking, it is important to organize the bedroom and remove any clutter in order to reduce the chance of falling. Also, it is important to lock all doors and windows in order to confine the sleepwalker to the bedroom.

You can put some small wind chimes up in the doorway in order to alert you when the sleepwalker is moving around.

When you encounter the sleepwalker, it is important to gently guide him back to their bed with a gentle, reassuring voice. Do not shake him, yell at him, or try to awaken him. He may misinterpret that as an attack and try to defend himself.

Remain calm. The sleepwalker usually responds well to stress-reduction techniques, relaxation techniques, good sleep hygiene, and a regular bedtime schedule. If the sleep walking continues or worsens, he or she may benefit from cognitive-behavioral therapy or counseling. Some may also benefit from targeted amino acid therapy, which uses amino acids to correct neurotransmitter imbalances. Visit www.neurorelief.com for more information.

Sleep-related eating disorder

This disorder affects up to 3 percent of the population. However, a higher percent, up to 15 percent, have an eating disorder. Sleep-related eating disorder typically involves sleepwalking and eating while asleep. Approximately, two-thirds of these patients are female, and approximately half are overweight.[19] They usually consume junk food and sweets but may eat cat food, dog food, or cookie dough. The medications Ambien and lithium may occasionally trigger this disorder. Also, stress, depression, eating disorders, personality

disorders, and insomnia may trigger this. However, elimi-
nating the triggering medications and stopping their sleepwalking will usually control the problem. Please follow the
instructions for sleepwalking.

Bruxism

Bruxism is simply grinding the teeth. This can ultimately
damage and destroy the teeth and also damage the TMJ,
which is the temporomandibular joint of the jaw. TMJ disorder is usually associated with severe pain in the jaw and
headaches. The pain can also be transferred to the ears or the
neck. The severe grinding of the teeth also typically awakens
the spouse. Approximately 8 percent of people grind their
teeth, and most are not even aware of it.[20]

To correct this problem, I usually refer my patients to a
dentist knowledgeable in bruxism and TMJ disorder in order
to fit them with a nocturnal bite splint, which protects their
teeth and jaw. I also refer them to a cognitive-behavioral
therapist and/or counseling as well as teach them stress-
reduction techniques and relaxation techniques. They also
usually benefit from good sleep hygiene, including a regular
bedtime schedule. I will also have them cut down on caffeine
and alcohol, especially in the afternoon and evening time.
Some of the supplements for insomnia are also beneficial for
those patients with bruxism.

REM sleep behavior disorder

This is a fairly rare parasomnia occurring in only about 0.5
percent of the population; the majority is older men, typically
over the age of sixty.[21]

This is a potentially dangerous disorder that can cause
harm to the patient or his spouse. It is typically due to a glitch

occurring with a mechanism that is supposed to paralyze the body during sleep; as the person dreams, he actually begins to act out his dreams. Occasionally the dreams are so intense that the person may injure himself or his spouse without even realizing it. The cause is unknown; however, certain medical conditions may precipitate it, including Parkinson's disease, dementia, some brain tumors and masses, and even narcolepsy.[22]

Patients with this disorder need to see a neurologist as well as a primary care physician for a comprehensive physical exam, neurological exam, and typically an MRI of the brain. Guns, knives, sharp objects, and all potentially dangerous objects should be removed from the bedroom. These patients usually need medication in order to control this potentially dangerous disorder. Good sleep hygiene—including a regular bedtime schedule—stress reduction, and relaxation exercises may also be beneficial.

Don't Lose Hope

Sleep disorders plague millions of people every day, the most common offender being insomnia, and while there may not be a cure-all for each one, there is absolutely no reason for you to lose hope that you will ever find rest. Many of these disorders can be treated naturally without drugs. The best thing is that you know what you are facing, because knowing is half the battle.

Building Blocks to a Better Night's Sleep

- Sleep disorders afflict an estimated sixty million Americans. Other reports state that 60 percent of American adults suffer from insomnia at least a few times each week. Are you part of the statistic?

- Sleep disorders fall into two categories—dyssomnias, which are connected to problems falling asleep and staying asleep, and parasomnias, which are behaviors that occur while sleeping.

- Secondary insomnia, which is a symptom rather than a cause, is far more common than primary insomnia.

- Just because you or someone you know snores doesn't necessarily mean sleep apnea is involved. Not everyone who snores has sleep apnea, but everyone who has sleep apnea snores.

Chapter 5

PROACTIVE SLEEP THERAPIES

E VERY PERSON AND animal in God's creation must
rest. The land and its plants rest as they cycle
through seasons. As a foundational principle of Creation, God designed rest to strengthen every aspect of your
life and health. The Bible says, "For thus says the Lord GOD,
the Holy One of Israel: 'In returning and rest you shall be
saved; in quietness and confidence shall be your strength'"
(Isa. 30:15).

Getting the rest you need is vital to everything you do.
Rest heals and restores your body, and rest in God saves or
delivers you from the pressures and stress that daily assault
your body and mind.

Let's take a look now at some sleep therapies that can get
you to sleep restfully without medication or those unpredict-
able side effects.

LIGHTEN THINGS UP

Believe it or not, how much bright sunlight you get during
the day can have a significant impact on how well you sleep.
Most Americans spend way too much time indoors with dim
artificial light or florescent lighting. Consequently we get far

too little bright sunlight. This disrupts our circadian clocks, which alters our mood, interferes with our sleep, and affects us both mentally and physically.

Low amounts of natural light exposure for a prolonged period of time may eventually cause an imbalance of the hormones serotonin and melatonin. This can lead to seasonal affective disorder, otherwise known as SAD. SAD involves experiencing a mild depression with symptoms of sadness, hopelessness, lethargy, weight loss or weight gain, and other symptoms of mild depression. This disorder usually occurs during late autumn and winter months when days grow shorter, thus limiting sunlight.

Also called winter depression, SAD affects about 11 million Americans each year.[1] These people need more sleep; they experience a decreased quality of sleep and wake up tired. Seasonal affective disorder is much more common in the northern part of the United States.

Getting enough sunlight during the day will help increase melatonin at night. It also helps to increase the neurotransmitters serotonin and norepinephrine. Melatonin and serotonin help to promote sleep, whereas norepinephrine and serotonin also help to elevate your mood.

Spend at least twenty to thirty minutes a day in the sunlight under a shade tree. If you live in the north where many days are overcast, it might help to purchase a light box that has full-spectrum lights. A much less expensive option is to simply purchase a light visor, which is simply a visor cap with LED lights on it. If you live in sunny southern climates where adequate sunlight is abundant, then sit outside at lunch for approximately thirty minutes under a shade tree or inside near a window that allows plenty of sunlight in and receive the healing power of light as you enjoy your lunch.[2]

If you work evenings, night shifts, or rotating shifts, a few changes may help—especially if you work rotating shifts. If you work at night and sleep during the day, be sure to sleep in a completely dark room with all light sealed out. Before you leave for work in the evening, spend time in a light box or wearing a light visor. Finally, when you return home in the morning, wear dark sunglasses that block out all light to prepare the mind and body for sleep.

GIVE YOURSELF A NAP

Research shows that people can increase alertness, reduce stress, and improve concentration and memory with a nap. A power nap also usually improves learning, improves reaction time, and makes you more patient, more efficient, and healthier.

Studies have shown that twenty minutes of sleep in the afternoon is significantly better than twenty minutes of more sleep in the morning. Sleep experts recommend that the nap be approximately twenty minutes in length. A nap longer than this will usually put you into a deeper stage of sleep, making you groggy and more difficult to awaken. Longer naps also actually interfere with sleep.

One study found that the short nap boosted performance by 34 percent and alertness by 54 percent.[3] A twenty-minute power nap in the early to mid-afternoon is a great way to boost energy, concentration, and memory, but do not get in the habit of using naps to make up for sleep debt, and do not take a nap if it prevents you from going to bed at your regular time.

Since so many Americans are sleep deprived, napping is one of the best ways for restoring and catching up on sleep.

A Behavioral Approach

To prevent insomnia, you usually need to learn methods to help you relax and fall asleep. There are numerous behavioral methods that do this. These behavioral techniques can relieve chronic insomnia in many cases. Many patients with primary insomnia are helped with behavioral therapy. Medications are equally as effective as behavioral therapy in helping people with insomnia.

However, most sleep medications are addictive, have side effects, and are unable to cure insomnia. Behavioral methods work fast and work in all age groups, including children as well as the elderly. The goal is simply to decrease the time it takes to fall to sleep to less than thirty minutes and also to decrease wakeup periods during the night. Of the patients treated with these nondrug methods, 70–80 percent have improved sleep, according to the studies. Even more amazing is that studies report that 75 percent of those taking medications to sleep are able to stop or reduce their use after having behavioral therapy.[4] I go into detail regarding many of these methods in my book *Stress Less*, but let's look at a few of the behavioral methods here.

Cognitive-behavioral therapy

Cognitive-behavioral therapy is a form of therapy that teaches patients how to recognize and change negative thought patterns and change the way they interpret events. It has been used in treating anxiety and depression for decades, but it is also very useful in treating insomnia. The patients with insomnia are commonly caught in negative thought patterns regarding sleep. Typical thoughts include:

- "I won't be able to fall asleep."
- "It will take me one or two hours to fall asleep."
- "I must get eight hours of sleep in order to function."
- "If I don't get enough sleep, my job performance will suffer greatly."

As a result of this negative thinking, they usually lie in bed unable to sleep. The treatment goal is to change their distortional thought patterns about their ability to fall asleep and stay asleep.

In Mark 11:24 Jesus said, "Therefore I say to you, whatever things you ask when you pray, believe that you receive them, and you will have them." If you believe that you won't be able to fall asleep or sleep through the night, then you won't be able to. However, we have a promise in Psalm 127:2 that says that God gives His beloved sleep. We are actually promised sleep in God's Word. Now, who are you going to side with—God's Word or your fears?

According to 2 Corinthians 10:4–5, it is critically important to tear down these mental strongholds, which are our fears and worries about sleep. Then begin to believe, confess, and visualize God giving His beloved—you!—sweet sleep. For more information on cognitive-behavioral therapy, please refer to my books *Stress Less* and *The New Bible Cure for Depression and Anxiety*. You can also find more information from the National Association of Cognitive-Behavioral Therapists at www.nacbt.org.

Progressive muscle relaxation

It takes about ten minutes to perform progressive muscle relaxation, which typically focuses on one muscle group at a time on one side of the body, usually starting in the feet. The muscles are tensed for five to ten seconds, and then the muscle is relaxed for about fifteen seconds. Then simply move up to the next muscle group and repeat the sequence for doing one side of the body at a time.

This technique was pioneered in the 1930s by Edmund Jacobson.[5] Jacobson believed that if people could learn to relax their muscles through a precise method, mental relaxation would follow. His technique involves tensing and relaxing various voluntary muscle groups throughout the body in an orderly sequence.[6]

Scientists today are learning the superior value this method of relaxation offers. According to psychologists Robert Woolfolk and Frank Richardson, "Despite the relative obscurity of this method, progressive relaxation is perhaps the most reliable and effective [relaxation] procedure of all."[7]

Progressive muscle relaxation (PMR), as it is called today, is one of the most simple and easily learned techniques for relaxation. It works because of the relationship between your muscle tension and your emotional tension; your emotional turmoil causes you to tense your muscles, unknowingly. That muscle tension causes other ailments, like headache and backache.

Do not begin this procedure without your doctor's evaluation. People who have had injuries, surgeries, or other ailments should not create tension in muscle groups that could cause further damage. I always recommend that you do no exercise program without your doctor's approval.

Dr. Colbert Approved — Bathe in Relaxation

Essential oils can be added directly to your bath water. Here's how:

- Add 5–10 drops of essential oils to hot water while filling your bath.
- Do not combine essential oils with other bath oils or soap.
- Make sure to soak in the tub for at least twenty minutes to get the aromatic benefits.

You can find essential oils at health food stores. The following essential oils have properties that are especially beneficial.

- Lavender. At first this oil may pep you up a little. But as you soak for a few minutes, you'll find that it calms you. It relieves nervous tension, depression, and insomnia.
- Geranium. Combine a couple drops of this with lavender. It has a calming effect.
- Rosemary. This one helps circulation. Use it alone or with lavender to relieve depression.
- Baking soda or Epsom salts. A hot bath in baking soda can do wonders for relaxing your muscles. Scoop a handful of baking soda or 1–2 cups of Epsom salts into very hot bath water and relax.

Abdominal breathing

Abdominal breathing is also known as diaphragmatic breathing. If you have ever gone to a newborn nursery, you will notice that all newborns are abdominal breathers. However, as we grow older and become more and more stressed, we eventually shift from being abdominal breathers to chest breathers. Chest breathing is stress breathing. However, opera singers and certain other professional singers, as well as musicians who play wind instruments, are usually abdominal breathers—and strengthening our abdominal breathing is one of the simplest, easiest, and best ways for us to decrease muscle tension, relax, and relieve stress, thus helping us sleep better.

Are you a chest or abdominal breather? To find out, simply lie on your back and place your right hand on your abdomen at your waistline (or on your belly button). Then place your left hand on the center of your chest. Now simply breathe normally and notice which hand rises more when you inhale. For most people, the hand on their chest will rise more. This means you are a chest breather. If the hand on your abdomen rises more, you are an abdominal breather.

To become an abdominal breather, you have to control your diaphragm, which is the muscle separating the chest cavity from the abdominal cavity. As you inhale, the diaphragm flattens downward, allowing the lungs more space to fill. By flattening this muscle, you allow more oxygen into the body and more carbon dioxide out of the body.

To do this, I recommend that you lie on your back on a bed, carpet, or rug. Put your legs straight out and mildly apart, with your toes pointed outward. Place one hand on your abdomen over the belly button and the other hand at the center of your chest. Slowly inhale through your nose, making sure the hand on the abdomen rises. Intentionally push out your abdomen; the hand on the chest should move only a little. As you inhale through your nose, count to yourself, "One thousand one, one thousand two, one thousand three." As you exhale through your mouth, count, "One thousand one, one thousand two, one thousand three." You should feel your abdomen falling as you exhale.

Some people take this exercise a step further. As they inhale, they say to themselves, "I breathe in the breath of relaxation," or they say, "Relaxation in" or "Peace in," to themselves. As they exhale, they say to themselves, "I breathe out tension," "I release the tension," "Tension out," or "Stress out."

Visualization

From our childhood we have discovered and developed the art of daydreaming. We used our imagination perhaps to escape the circumstances we were in or to dream of what we would like to be or do. Unfortunately, as our minds become more active and fretful over many things, our imaginations become more negative and corrupt. People imagine catastrophes that will come to them and many kinds of unclean thoughts, all of which can keep us from a restful mode of life. But using our imagination in a healthy way can be a useful technique for relaxation.

We all practice mental visualization on a daily basis, even if we're not aware that we do. Daydreaming and imagining are visualization techniques. There is great benefit in reducing stress by purposefully and consciously using visualization techniques.

Find a quiet place where you will not be disturbed, and

lie down or sit in a comfortable chair. Think of an image, place, memory, or scene that relaxes you. Allow yourself to be immersed in your image by involving all five senses in the visualization. See the images, hear the sounds, feel the fabric or air temperature, smell and taste items related to your image, and so forth.

If your favorite vacation spot is the beach, imagine yourself walking along the beach on a bright, sunny day, experiencing the ocean breeze as it blows through your hair, the warmth of the sun on your skin, and hearing the slap of the waves on the shoreline; taste the salty air, and breathe deeply the relaxation all of that brings. Let your imagination be filled with the sights, sounds, and other comforting sensory perceptions you have experienced. Whatever your relaxing daydream is, spend five or ten minutes there, and see what relaxation effects it has on your psyche. And don't forget to return to mindful thoughts about the blessings of the present moment.

Meditation

Meditation is also beneficial as a behavioral technique for insomnia. In essence, it involves a process of focusing one's attention on only one thing at a time and letting all other thoughts go. Simply put, meditation is "focused thinking." If a stray thought comes to a meditating person's mind, he should not resist that thought or judge it—rather, he should simply notice it and then immediately let it go. The conscious mind should remain focused on a word or phrase that the person has chosen to focus on through repetition.

God promised a prosperous life of success for those who would quietly meditate on the Word of God continually. While there are many forms of meditation, my favorite is meditating on Scripture. You may call this reflecting on God's Word or contemplating God's Word. It doesn't take great skill to learn to meditate, just a decision to become quiet, control your thoughts, and center in on one idea. What better ideas than what the Word of God offers?

According to Rick Warren, the author of *The Purpose-Driven Life*, "If you know how to worry, you already know how to meditate."[8] Worry is also focused thinking—focusing on the problem. In meditation, the goal is to help a person gain and sustain a positive focus. For the Christian, what a person focuses upon is just as important as the focusing technique.

The unnecessary stressors this culture presses upon us can be overcome as we choose to meditate on God's Word. Jesus said, "The words that I speak to you are spirit, and they are life" (John 6:63). I choose especially to focus on the words of Jesus as I meditate. I repeat what I have memorized of the words of Jesus as I sit calmly. I train my mind to focus on His words, and I allow them to sink deep into my heart and soul.

Biofeedback

Biofeedback teaches how to control physiologic functions such as muscle tension, heart rate, breathing, blood pressure, skin temperature, perspiration, and even brain waves through the use of instruments and machines. Each of these biological parameters can be controlled to some extent by working with a biofeedback trainer. By learning to control these functions, you can usually learn to improve your sleep.

There are actually four different types of biofeedback: neurofeedback, EMG biofeedback, respiratory biofeedback, and thermal biofeedback. I find that neurofeedback and EMG biofeedback especially are beneficial to my patients with insomnia.

In a biofeedback session a person works with a trained professional to identify which aspects of the nervous system are not relaxed. For example, a person's EEG may show alpha wave activity in the brain (a sign of relaxation), but the EMG shows muscle tension and the skin temperature is cool—both are signs of stress. Biofeedback helps a person identify what aspect of the body needs to be addressed with a relaxation technique.

Most large cities and major universities offer biofeedback training. To find a certified biofeedback practitioner, call (303) 422–8436. Some companies offer less expensive home biofeedback "trainers" that can be hooked up to a person's computer. You might ask a certified practitioner about these programs to determine which is best for you. Again, biofeedback is not a relaxation technique, per se. Rather, it is helpful in learning where and how to focus relaxation techniques.

MASSAGE IT OUT

There are at least two hundred known massage techniques. From perhaps the oldest, acupressure, dating back five thousand years, to those forms of massage developed in the twentieth century, these techniques do benefit the relaxation process of the body and can certainly help you sleep better at night. Massage is always a recommendation I give my patients, especially if their condition is exacerbated by stress.

Even a handheld massage device can help to relieve tension in the muscles, thereby relieving stress. There are even massages that accommodate our hectic "airport" routines. The "chair massage" is designed to relax you as you are massaged in a special chair, fully clothed, waiting for your next flight. You could even invite a practitioner to bring his or her portable massage chair to your office or business, or to a party for your invited guests' benefit. This ten- or twenty-minute massage can bring moderate relaxation, wherever it is administered.[9]

The Bowen Technique is named after Australian Tom Bowen, who in the 1950s introduced the concept of having rest periods between a series of massage movements, allowing the body to absorb the healing process before continuing the session. This technique involves gentle, soft tissue manipulations, which are precise and intended to create harmony within the body, allowing it to make its own adjustments and achieve its own cure.[10] This type of massage is able to balance the autonomic nervous system, relieving stress significantly. I routinely prescribe this type of massage for my patients.

REAP THE BENEFITS

Taking advantage of sleep therapies to retrain your body's internal clock or to change negative thoughts toward sleep will benefit you in more ways than one. You will find that these strategies will spill over into other parts of your life, creating a stress-free, peaceful, and balanced existence. Follow up on the details for many of these strategies in my books *Stress Less* and *The New Bible Cure for Depression and Anxiety* to really see the far-reaching, lifelong benefits you can attain.

Building Blocks to a Better Night's Sleep

- It's as important to get sunlight as it is to reduce the light once nighttime comes.

- Your mind carries a lot of power over your ability to sleep. Practice cognitive-behavioral therapy, progressive muscle relaxation, abdominal breathing, visualization, and meditation to help yourself get better rest.

Chapter 6

HEALTHY LIFESTYLE CHANGES FOR A BETTER NIGHT'S SLEEP

NOT ONLY DID God create the world to be founded upon a principle of rest, but He also created a dynamic display of delicious fruits, vegetables, and many other foods to provide you with a wonderful array of nutritious choices. All that your body needs for divine health and rest has been bountifully provided for you by your loving heavenly Father. It's no wonder the psalmist declared, "Return to your rest, O my soul, for the LORD has dealt bountifully with you" (Ps. 116:7).

Learning how to use God's wisdom in giving your body the right nutritional selections can be a mighty key in breaking the power of sleep disorders and finding rest for your weary body and soul.

Let's take a look at how nutrition can help you.

REST IN WHAT YOU EAT

What you eat and what you don't eat are major keys in how well you sleep, for nutrition and sleep are very much related. You wouldn't put water into your gas tank and expect your car to run, would you? Your car needs to be fueled properly, according to its design. Well, the designer of your body, God, has provided just the right fuel for you!

> And God said, "See, I have given you every herb that yields seed which is on the face of all the earth, and every tree whose fruit yields seed; to you it shall be for food. Also, to every beast of the earth, to every bird of the air, and to everything that creeps on the earth, in which there is life, I have given every green herb for food"; and it was so. Then God saw everything that He had made, and indeed it was very good.
> —GENESIS 1:29–31

If your diet contains excessive sugar, fat, starch, and salt, you are probably experiencing fatigue and even chronic fatigue. Balanced nutrition helps your body fight off fatigue and sustains you through demanding and stressful situations.

Breakfast first

When a person awakens in the morning, his blood sugar is generally low because he hasn't eaten for eight to twelve hours. What a person eats for breakfast is extremely important. The typical American breakfast consists of coffee and a bagel or doughnut. Or it may be a glass of juice with a bowl of cereal or pancakes, waffles, pastry, or toast. These high-sugar, high-carb foods generally lead to hypoglycemia. They are precisely the wrong foods to eat!

The bread and white-flour items I listed above are all foods that convert quickly into sugar. Juice is very high in sugar. Orange, grape, and apple juices are all high in fructose, a fruit sugar. Grapefruit juice and cranberry juice are better choices, but even then, I recommend only 4 ounces of juice or less. It is far better to choose whole fruits. The whole fruit is less likely to raise insulin levels.

Many people skip breakfast and eat a small lunch, then have a large dinner in the evening. I find this is very common among my patients, and especially among my stressed-out and overweight patients.

If you skip breakfast, you will have fasted (gone without food) for twelve to sixteen or more hours by the time you eat lunch. You probably have put your body into a temporary hypoglycemic state by that time. Every time you do this, your adrenals are stimulated to produce more cortisol and your cravings for sugar and carbohydrates will increase. By the time a person reaches the dinner hour, that person will most likely have experienced many episodes of "hypoglycemia" during the day since they likely have snacked on sugar and highly processed carbohydrate foods. Their insulin levels are usually elevated, and they are in "fat-storage" mode.

While in this fat-storage mode, they eat a large dinner with bread, meat, a vegetable, a starch, and a dessert! They go to bed a couple of hours later. The elevated insulin tells the body to store the sugars and carbohydrates as glycogen in the liver and muscles, and the excess carb and sugar calories as fat. So the person awakens the next morning having "stored" all that excess food. And the process begins all over again.

How then should a person eat? A person ideally should eat mainly low-glycemic carbohydrates balanced with healthy fats and lean, free-range, or organic protein foods. A person should "graze" throughout the day, eating three well-balanced meals and two to three smaller and well-balanced snacks—one between breakfast and lunch, one between lunch and dinner, and sometimes a bedtime snack.

For years I have told my patients to eat breakfast like a king, lunch like a prince, and dinner like a pauper. The most important meal of the day is breakfast. By choosing the right foods in proper balance at breakfast, as well as other meals, a person can greatly lower his or her insulin and cortisol levels to normal and greatly assist any weight-loss plan.

Dr. Colbert's Protein Smoothie

DR. COLBERT APPROVED

Here's a delicious protein smoothie that you can enjoy at bedtime. Not only will it help you to balance your blood sugar, but it will also improve your health as well.

- 1 scoop protein powder (Life's Basics protein, whey, or rice protein, equal to 14–15 g protein)
- 1–2 Tbsp. of ground flaxseeds
- ¼–½ cup frozen strawberries, raspberries, blackberries, or blueberries, or a combination of them OR
- ½ frozen banana
- 1 cup water, coconut milk or kefir, or organic skim milk or kefir

Blend into a smoothie and enjoy!

Protein matters

A simple way to calculate your protein requirement is to take your weight in pounds and divide it by two. That is the amount of protein a person should have per day in grams.

As an example, if a person weighs 170 pounds, he needs 85 grams of protein a day.

Men generally need no more than 4 to 5 ounces of protein per meal, and women 3 to 4 ounces per meal. Men can generally eat 5 to 8 ounces of fish at a meal, and women 4 to 6 ounces.

Choose the leanest piece of meat you can, with little or no marbling, and trim off any visible fat. It is important to peel off the skin and cut away any visible fat from chicken and poultry. Choose white meat rather than dark meat. Grill, bake, or broil your meats rather than frying them. If you grill your food, be sure to avoid charred meats since they contain a chemical called benzopyrene, which is carcinogenic (cancer causing). I strongly advise against deep-frying any food since these fats create a tremendous amount of free radicals in the body. Free radicals are highly reactive molecules that damage cells and tissues. They are produced in the body and have an unpaired electron in their outer field. If you must fry a food, lightly stir-fry it at the lowest temperature possible, with a little organic butter or cold-pressed macadamia nut oil. Macadamia nut oil is better than olive oil for frying since its smoke point is greater than four hundred degrees Fahrenheit, whereas olive oil's smoke point is only about two hundred degrees Fahrenheit. You can find cold-pressed macadamia nut oil at most health food stores.

I also recommend that you limit or avoid highly processed meats such as hot dogs, bologna, sausage, cold cuts, ham, bacon, and most packaged luncheon meats. They are generally very high in sodium content, very high in fat, and usually have nitrites and nitrates added. Nitrites and nitrates are converted in the digestive tract to nitrosamines, which are associated with an increased risk of cancer.

Carbs can be good

Not all carbohydrates are bad—a person needs a sufficient quantity of "good" carbohydrates. Proteins, fats, and carbohydrates need to be in the right balance. Understanding which carbohydrates have a favorable glycemic index is a key to preventing hypoglycemia and keeping insulin and cortisol levels normal.

High-glycemic carbohydrates—which are rapidly converted to sugar—may cause an insulin spike. A large quantity of medium glycemic index carbohydrates can also cause a spike. It is best to stick to low glycemic index foods and to greatly curtail those that are high or even moderately high glycemic.

Low-glycemic carbohydrates include most green vegetables such as lettuce, zucchini, squash, spinach, cabbage, and so on. It also includes low-glycemic fruits such as berries, kiwi, Granny Smith apples, and grapefruit. Whole grains rich in soluble fiber are also low glycemic and include old-fashioned oatmeal (not instant), oat bran, and other high-fiber foods.

High-glycemic carbohydrates include starches and most processed grains (such as white breads, processed pastas, and white rice), starchy vegetables (such as potatoes and corn), and high-glycemic fruits (such as dried fruits). For more information on this topic, refer to *The New Bible Cure for Weight Loss*.

Not all fat is bad

Fats are extremely important for good health. They help form cell membranes and regulate what enters and exits the cells. They are a critical part of most body tissues. More than 60 percent of the dry weight of the brain is fat!

Fat forms the myelin sheath in nerve cells, which is similar to electrical wire insulation. Fat is required for the synapses or connections between the nerves, which allow information to be transmitted. Fat forms the building blocks for the body's pro- and anti-inflammatory compounds.

The important thing about dietary fat is this: not all fats are created equal! Healthy fats include the omega-3 and omega-9 fats.

Omega-3 fats supply the building blocks for powerful anti-inflammatory compounds in the body. Alpha-linolenic acid is a powerful omega-3 fat that is found in flaxseed and dark green leafy vegetables. The most potent omega-3 fat is eicosapentaenoic acid (EPA), which is found in cold-water fish and fish oils (which may be taken as supplements in capsule form). This omega-3 fat assists in the body's production of inflammation-suppressing substances. High-quality fish oil has been linked to significant reduction of inflammation in the body.[1]

Fish with the highest concentrations of omega-3 oils are mackerel, Pacific herring, king salmon, Atlantic salmon, anchovies, and lake trout. Wild salmon contains higher omega-3 fat than farm-raised salmon.

Monounsaturated fats, which are the omega-9 fats, have no direct effect on insulin or inflammation, but they are still considered very healthy fats. These fats include olive oil (extra virgin is preferred), avocado, and nut oils—including almond and macadamia nut. I personally enjoy extra-virgin olive oil and balsamic vinegar as a salad dressing. I recommend that you use almond butter in place of peanut butter for omega-9 benefit.

Use these omega-9 fats in moderation, and they will help create the correct fuel mixture to lower both insulin and cortisol levels.

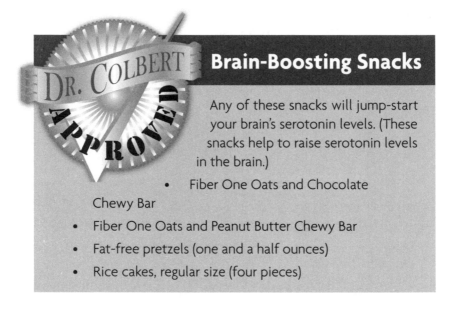

DR. COLBERT APPROVED

Brain-Boosting Snacks

Any of these snacks will jump-start your brain's serotonin levels. (These snacks help to raise serotonin levels in the brain.)

- Fiber One Oats and Chocolate Chewy Bar
- Fiber One Oats and Peanut Butter Chewy Bar
- Fat-free pretzels (one and a half ounces)
- Rice cakes, regular size (four pieces)

SUPPLEMENT YOUR FOOD

To begin a supplementation program, I strongly recommend a comprehensive multivitamin and multimineral supplement that contains adequate levels of B vitamins, magnesium, and trace minerals. This will provide optimal nutritional supplementation for a good night's sleep.

Several special herbs and other supplements are especially effective in helping you sleep. However, you will find that supplementing with magnesium, melatonin, certain amino acids, herbs, or hormones at bedtime, or drinking teas, is very effective; also, these teas and supplements are nonaddictive, unlike most medications for sleep. Herbs and supplements for sleep are usually used on a short-term basis unless you have anxiety, depression, or a deficiency in melatonin or certain calming neurotransmitters.

Let's look at some of these helpful supplements.

Melatonin

Melatonin is a hormone produced by a small gland, called the pineal gland, in the brain. Melatonin helps to regulate sleep and wake cycles, or circadian rhythms. Usually melatonin begins to rise in the evening and remains high for most of the night and then decreases in the early morning. Melatonin production is affected by light. As a person ages, melatonin levels decline. Older adults typically produce very small amounts of melatonin or none at all. Studies suggest that melatonin induces sleep without suppressing REM or dream sleep, whereas most sleep meds suppress REM sleep.[2]

Melatonin works best if the patient's melatonin levels are low. Children generally have normal levels of melatonin; therefore, supplementation with melatonin in children usually is ineffective. However, in adults, especially the elderly, it may be very effective in treating insomnia and is excellent in treating jet lag. It is also usually very effective for those who work the night shift.

The main side effect of melatonin is sleepiness, which is good; however, other potential side effects include vivid dreams, morning grogginess, and headaches. The recommended dose of melatonin is typically 1–6 mg at bedtime. I recommend a melatonin lozenge since it dissolves in the mouth and seems to work better for most patients. I start my patients on a low dose and gradually increase the dose until the patient is sleeping well. I also commonly continue melatonin with other natural sleep aids that you will be soon learning about. Remember, melatonin as well as other sleep aids work best when practicing good sleep hygiene.

DR. COLBERT APPROVED

Adrenal Glandular Supplements

Glandular therapy has been used for thousands of years, all the way back to ancient Egypt. Today, products like Armour Thyroid are still quite popular in treating patients with hypothyroidism (low thyroid function). Adrenal glandular supplements contain protomorphogens or extracts of tissues from the adrenal glands of pigs or cattle. These can be taken orally to support human adrenal function. Glandular substances in pigs and cattle have an "adrenal mix" close to that of the human adrenal glands. Some doctors of natural medicine have used adrenal glandular supplements with their patients for decades and report very positive results.

L-tryptophan and 5-HTP (5-hydroxytryptophan)

I commonly place patients with insomnia on melatonin and the amino acid L-tryptophan or 5-HTP. L-tryptophan improves sleep normalcy and increases stage four sleep (the most restorative stage of sleep). It has also been shown to improve obstructive sleep apnea in many patients, and it does not decrease cognitive performance.

Both L-tryptophan and its metabolite 5-HTP are used to increase serotonin levels in the brain. Serotonin is a neurotransmitter in the brain that promotes restful sleep and well-being as well as satiety.

However, when serotonin levels are low in the brain, you are more prone to experience insomnia. Serotonin levels are also increased by ingesting carbohydrates. When carbohydrates are ingested with L-tryptophan or 5-HTP, the elevated insulin level increases the removal of other amino acids that compete with tryptophan and 5-HTP for transport into the brain. Carbohydrates also tend to increase the sedative effects of 5-HTP and tryptophan.

I recommend vitamin B$_6$, niacin, and magnesium, which serve as cofactors in the conversion of L-tryptophan and 5-HTP to serotonin. I usually recommend simply taking either 1,000–2,000 mg of L-tryptophan or 100–300 mg of 5-HTP at bedtime. In addition, I recommend a comprehensive multivitamin that contains adequate amounts of vitamin B$_6$, niacin, and magnesium, which helps convert L-tryptophan and 5-HTP to serotonin. Also, I usually have the patients take their L-tryptophan or 5-HTP with a food that is high in carbohydrate and low in protein.

L-theanine and GABA

I have found that most patients with insomnia are under excessive stress and may be suffering from anxiety and depression. Excessive stress, anxiety, and depression are usually associated with elevated cortisol levels, especially at night. Elevated stress hormones, especially cortisol, eventually disrupt brain chemistry, causing imbalances in neurotransmitters, including serotonin, dopamine, norepinephrine, and GABA, as well as other brain chemicals.

However, the amino acid L-theanine crosses the blood-brain

barrier and is able to suppress stress hormones, including cortisol. L-theanine is one of the natural chemicals found in green tea and helps to decrease stress and anxiety. It also helps the body produce other calming neurotransmitters, including GABA, serotonin, and dopamine. In Japan L-theanine is usually added to sodas and chewing gum to provide a relaxing and soothing effect.[3]

I find that L-theanine typically works better with the amino acid GABA. GABA is also a calming neurotransmitter in the brain that has a soothing effect on the nervous system. L-theanine and GABA supplements taken with vitamin B_6 usually help to calm the mind as well as lower the stress hormones and help you fall asleep. I usually recommend 200–400 mg of L-theanine with 500–1,000 mg of GABA at bedtime taken with a comprehensive multivitamin containing vitamin B_6. This combination may also be taken with melatonin and 5-HTP or L-tryptophan. For more information on GABA, please see *The New Bible Cure for Depression and Anxiety*.

Magnesium

We already know that adequate amounts of magnesium are needed to help convert L-tryptophan and 5-HTP to serotonin. There is also a close association between normal sleep architecture and magnesium. The excitatory neurotransmitter glutamate disrupts normal sleep architecture, causing insomnia, whereas the inhibitory neurotransmitter GABA usually improves sleep architecture. Magnesium is a mineral that helps decrease the glutamate activity in the brain while at the same time increasing the GABA activity in the brain.

This usually helps to improve sleep. Thus, magnesium is able to help many patients with insomnia issues.

I commonly recommend a magnesium powder, Natural Calm, to patients with insomnia. Simply taking 1½ teaspoons of Natural Calm in 4 ounces of hot water as a tea at bedtime provides 307 mg of magnesium and helps many of my patients fall asleep.

Other teas to treat insomnia

For centuries people have used chamomile tea to treat insomnia. Chamomile tea is a mild muscle relaxant and has mild sedative properties; it may also help relieve stress, anxiety, and depression. It usually helps promote a deep sleep as well as feelings of relaxation and calmness. The active ingredients are volatile oils found in the flowers of chamomile.

Sleepytime Tea blends floral Egyptian chamomile with cool spearmint from the Pacific Northwest and Guatemalan lemongrass. Another tea called Tilo, also known as linden flower tea, has gentle relaxing properties that help to relieve stress and may help relieve anxiety. In choosing teas, always choose organic teas. Many of my patients use these teas as sleep aids and have found them to be very beneficial in treating insomnia. However, a word of caution: people who are allergic to ragweed should avoid chamomile and Sleepytime Tea.

Valerian root

Valerian root is another herb that has been used for many years for insomnia; it also helps to calm the mind. It is believed that valerian works by increasing GABA levels in the brain. With its mild sedative qualities valerian helps people fall asleep and improve their quality of sleep. It may take two to three weeks to appreciate its full effect. Valerian root may

DR. COLBERT APPROVED

Teas to Help You Sleep

If you're having trouble falling asleep, try drinking a cup of Celestial Seasonings Sleepytime Extra Wellness Tea or Yogi Bedtime Tea one to two hours before bedtime. These are all-natural, no-caffeine herbal teas. Sleepytime Tea contains chamomile, tilia estella, and 25 mg of valerian. Yogi Bedtime Tea contains organic skullcap leaf. However, do not give these teas to children. If you are pregnant, nursing, or on medications, consult with your physician before drinking the tea.

be taken as pills or tea; however, the tea has a very unpleasant taste. If you choose any herbal supplement including valerian, make sure it is organic.

Unlike medications, no standard dosing guidelines have been established for valerian root. For treating insomnia, a valerian root dosage that is sometimes recommended is 300–900 mg per day. It's best to take it thirty minutes to two hours before bedtime.

Magnolia bark and adaptogens

Magnolia bark, *magnolia officinalis,* a traditional Chinese medicine, has been used for thousands of years to help with low energy, emotional distress, digestive problems, diarrhea, and more. Modern research has focused on magnolia for its sedative and muscle relaxant properties. Magnolia especially helps patients who are under a lot of stress or who suffer from anxiety.

Adaptogens are substances that help the body adapt to stress by balancing the adrenal glands' response to stress. Adaptogens include rhodiola, ashwagandha, ginseng, and many more. Since excessive stress is a major cause of insomnia, adaptogens given in the evening may be effective in calming the mind and body. For more information on adaptogens, refer to my book *Stress Less*.

Progesterone

Numerous studies have shown that over 50 percent of all perimenopausal and postmenopausal women have problems falling asleep or staying asleep.[4] This is commonly due to fluctuating levels or low levels of estrogen and progesterone. We also know that women experiencing hot flashes and night sweats usually have a poorer quality of sleep. Bioidentical hormone therapy is one of the simplest yet most profound ways to improve sleep in perimenopausal and postmenopausal women.

Estrogen has an excitatory effect on the brain, whereas progesterone has a calming and soothing effect on the brain. Women with estrogen dominance, which is common prior to menopause, usually experience restless sleep, whereas progesterone replacement usually dramatically improves sleep. Studies show that progesterone has antianxiety effects by stimulating GABA receptors in the brain.[5] This in turn helps you relax and sleep. GABA also helps balance excitation with inhibition. Researchers have found that progesterone produces a sleep brain wave pattern similar to that of tranquilizers.[6]

I usually check hormone levels in women with insomnia and commonly find low progesterone levels. I check the serum progesterone on day twenty-one of their menstrual cycle. Then I start them on 100 mg of bioidentical progesterone (not synthetic progesterone) at bedtime. Progesterone also must be balanced with bioidentical estrogen. To find a physician who is knowledgeable about bioidentical hormone replacement therapy, refer to www.worldhealth.net.

I want to emphasize that herbs and supplementation should usually be used on a short-term basis unless you have anxiety or depression or if you are over the age of fifty and are deficient in melatonin.

Supplements for Sleep Disorders

Since so many sleep disorders exist, let's look beyond insomnia to some supplements that help relieve the less-common sleep disorders.

Restless legs syndrome

If you are experiencing restless legs syndrome, get your doctor to test you to see if your body is low in iron. A test called a ferritin level blood test can measure the iron stores in your body. If your ferritin level is low, supplementing with iron may relieve restless legs syndrome.

Regular aerobic exercise, leg massages, and warm baths with Epsom salts, 1 to 4 cups in the bathwater, can also help relieve the symptoms of restless legs syndrome. Also supplementation with magnesium at bedtime may help. See suggested dosage of magnesium on the next page.

Periodic limb movement disorder

Periodic limb movement disorder is another movement disorder associated with insomnia. This involuntary disorder often causes repetitive, jerking twitches of the legs that last between one and three seconds. This twitching can wake up the sleeper or his or her spouse. Those with this disorder tend to feel quite drowsy throughout the day.

Here are some supplements that may help:

- 400 mg of magnesium in the form of magnesium citrate, magnesium aspartate, or magnesium glycinate OR

- 1–2 tsp. of Natural Calm in 4 oz. of hot water at bedtime

In addition, taking a warm bath and adding 1–4 cups of Epsom salts to the bathwater may also help.

Exercise to Help You Rest

Most people think they exercise for the sake of their body—generally to stay lean and strong physically. The greater truth is that exercise is also good for the mind and emotions.

The benefits of exercise are far-reaching. They are not only "external" in the form of appearance, flexibility, and manifestations of strength. They are also "internal" at the cellular level. Several types of exercises are directly related to stress reduction and can help prepare your mind and body for a good night's sleep.

Those who exercise regularly also spend a greater amount of time in stage three and stage four sleep, which are the most restorative, repairing stages of sleep. By spending more time in stages three and four sleep, you will awaken more refreshed and have much more energy throughout the day. However, don't exercise within three to four hours of bedtime, for this can actually cause insomnia.

Aerobic exercise

Aerobic exercise is one of the best ways to improve the quality of your sleep. It helps you to fall asleep faster and to sleep longer. *Aerobic* literally means "in the presence of air." Aerobic exercises increase the oxygen-carrying capacity of the body as a whole. The muscles and cardiovascular system both become stronger and more efficient if a person is exercising aerobically on a regular basis.

Aerobic exercises are generally those that exercise the large muscle groups of the body in repetitive motions for a sustained period of time. Such exercises include brisk walking, jogging, cycling, swimming, rowing, aerobic dance routines, stair stepping, skating, and cross-country skiing. Active sports, such as singles tennis, racquetball, and basketball, also produce an aerobic effect.

Aerobic exercise has been shown in countless studies to decrease the risk of cardiovascular disease and cancer, decrease body weight, lower blood pressure, and lower triglycerides and LDL (bad) cholesterol. It also helps raise HDL (good) cholesterol, helps prevent diabetes, and improves glucose tolerance. It increases a person's energy level and promotes more restful sleep.

Aerobic exercise increases the release of endorphins and norepinephrine in the brain. Endorphins are hormone-like substances that elevate mood and give a person a sense of well-being. In this way, aerobic exercise has an antidepressant effect. You may have heard of something called a "runner's high"—those who exercise vigorously and regularly often feel euphoric as they exercise. They are getting "high" on their own release of endorphins.

Moderate aerobic exercise reduces cortisol levels, but aerobic exercise that is too intense or prolonged may raise cortisol levels. Few people need to worry about whether they are exercising too intensely or for too lengthy a period—the vast majority of people don't get enough aerobic exercise.

The greatest benefits of aerobic exercise tend to occur if a person exercises early in the morning. This is especially true if a person is attempting to lose weight. However, the time a person does aerobic exercise is not nearly as important as the frequency and duration of the exercise—just be sure not to exercise within three to four hours of going to sleep. A person should do aerobic exercises three to four times a week for twenty to thirty minutes each time.

Add stretching and resistance

It is important to add stretching exercises as well as resistance exercises, also called weight training, to your aerobic exercise. Stretching exercises can help relieve tension and loosen uptight, tense muscles. Stretching promotes flexibility and can help greatly in reducing injuries. It also helps reduce symptoms of arthritis. Stretches are simple to do, but they should be accompanied by proper breathing techniques.

It is best to stretch muscles after they are warm—in other words, after you have done some aerobic exercising. Exercising a cold muscle is like pulling a rubber band that has been in the refrigerator and isn't warm. An optimal approach for reducing musculoskeletal injuries is to walk for ten minutes

DR. COLBERT APPROVED

Find Your Target Heart Rate Zone

I used to recommend purchasing a heart rate monitor or calculating your target heart rate zone by using a formula I provided, but most modern exercise equipment now has a heart rate monitor feature built in. However, if you don't have access to such equipment, I have a very simple solution. To find your target heart rate zone, simply walk fast enough so that you can't sing and slow enough so that you can talk. If you are walking so fast that you can't carry on a conversation, slow down. But if you are walking so slow that you are able to sing, speed up.

Also, find a buddy who is close to your fitness level. I have seen spouses walking in my neighborhood, and the husband is way ahead of the wife. The poor wife is huffing and puffing, trying to catch up. This will add more stress to your life because exercise should be enjoyable and not a chore.

at a moderate pace, stop to do a series of stretching exercises for fifteen minutes, and then continue with more vigorous walking for twenty minutes. Give your muscles a cool-down period of another five minutes of relaxed walking.

Never stretch a muscle to the point where you feel prolonged pain. At the first sign of pain, back off to a "stretch point" where you feel no pain.

Resistance exercises are also very important to preserve muscle mass and prevent osteoporosis. You can benefit greatly in this by joining a gym, going regularly, and working with a certified personal trainer who can help you set weights and develop a program that is right for you.

Alternative forms of exercise

A number of alternate forms of exercise also have been shown to have excellent benefits in reducing stress and improving overall health. Although as a believer I don't condone the practice of Eastern religions, I do, however, believe the various forms of exercise that they have introduced to the Western world are highly beneficial to most people. If people only knew how helpful these exercises can be in overcoming stress and other health issues, they would be less likely to label it a taboo subject. We can participate in the exercises and breathing techniques without getting involved with the religion.

Yoga

Yoga is a form of exercise that combines stretching and breathing to relax the body.

There are several types of yoga. "Hatha" yoga is the most popular type practiced in the United States. More than eighteen million Americans now practice yoga, which is up from six million people just a decade or so ago.[7]

Yoga is more than five thousand years old and is an ancient Eastern practice initially designed to bring the body, mind, and soul into harmony. It was and is considered an alternate form of physical activity. Yoga is "low impact," and Hatha yoga concentrates on these three activities: controlled breathing, posture, and meditation. The slow breathing promotes relaxation, and the various "postures" of yoga promote flexibility by gently stretching the body into different positions.

Yoga is different from most other forms of exercise in that

it is not concerned with how many repetitions are performed or how well a person performs a particular exercise. Instead, yoga focuses a person's attention on how the body is structured and how to move the body without aggravating an injury or causing pain. It teaches a person how to breathe properly and how to integrate breathing with positions of the body. A person doesn't strain or "force" the body in doing yoga, but rather, gently stretches various muscles. With practice, yoga can improve a person's strength, flexibility, endurance, and help reduce stress. A recent study reported in the *Journal of the American Medical Association* reported that daily yoga practice could reduce the pain associated with carpal tunnel syndrome.[8]

Tai Chi

Tai Chi is an ancient Chinese martial art that involves slow, smooth, and fluid movements. As a martial art, Tai Chi has been practiced for many centuries.

Tai Chi emphasizes diaphragmatic or abdominal breathing. Research has shown that Tai Chi may improve muscle mass, tone, flexibility, strength, stamina, balance, coordination, posture, and well-being. It can also provide similar cardiovascular benefits to modern aerobic exercise.

One of the most beneficial effects of Tai Chi is its ability to reduce stress. The regular practice of Tai Chi was shown in one study to increase noradrenaline excretion in the urine, as well as to decrease salivary cortisol concentrations. These two effects are directly related to the lowering of stress. Subjects reported feeling less tension, depression, anger, fatigue, confusion, and anxiety, and they felt more vigorous.[9]

Tai Chi is practiced slowly with smooth, low-intensity, graceful movements, which are accompanied by rhythmic abdominal breathing. A typical exercise session is a series of gentle, deliberate moves or postures combined into a sequential "choreography" of sorts. These movements are called "forms," and each form has between twenty and one hundred moves. The exercise typically requires up to twenty minutes to complete a basic form. Tai Chi relies totally on technique rather than power or strength.

Tai Chi lowers stress hormones, reduces tension, increases energy, and helps clear the mind. It can be practiced by a person at any age and by individuals who have a wide range of chronic diseases. The calming effect of Tai Chi changes the brain's frequency from "beta," which is the normal waking wave pattern, to "alpha," which is associated with an improved ability to learn and remember. Tai Chi calms the mind, promotes flexibility, and exercises and tones the body, including the cardiovascular system—all at the same time. Tai Chi, like yoga, includes meditation. However, I encourage my patients to practice the exercise and to only meditate on God's Word.

Mix it up

Find a good balance of regular exercise that is tailored to your fitness level, sleep pattern, nutritional status, weight, stress level, and busy schedule. Make it personal, and make it fun! A variety of exercises can help keep you motivated.

I advise my patients to schedule a workout at least every other day and to put that workout time in their appointment book—and then keep the appointment, just as if they were making an appointment with a physician or a business consultant. I also encourage my patients to have a "training partner" to whom they are accountable for sticking with a regular exercise program. On days when you are simply too exhausted or too stressed, or after nights in which you have not slept well, don't push yourself to exercise. Listen to your body, and learn when to exercise and when to rest.

Keep in mind, however, that an exercise program that includes a balance of stretching, resistance, and aerobic exercises will do far more to reduce stress than choosing not to exercise at all. Even people with severe fatigue benefit from mild exercise, such as stretching and a leisurely walk.

IT'S ABOUT WISDOM

The promise of living wisely includes enjoying the benefits of refreshing, restoring sweet sleep. Dragging through your days fatigued and tossing through your nights awake is not healthy or wise.

But knowledge and wisdom are really never far away from any one of us. As a matter of fact, the Bible says that wisdom is everywhere—we just need to open our ears and hear it. The Word of God says, "Wisdom calls aloud outside; she raises her voice in the open squares. She cries out in the chief concourses, at the openings of the gates in the city.... 'Turn at my rebuke; surely I will pour out my spirit on you; I will make my words known to you'" (Prov. 1:20–21, 23).

Why not simply ask God to give you a wise and understanding heart?

Building Blocks to a Better Night's Sleep

- A healthy lifestyle that promotes rest includes good eating habits, nutrition, and exercise.

- It's true—breakfast really is the most important meal of the day.

- Natural supplements to aid in sleep are far superior to prescription or over-the-counter sleep aids. Choose melatonin, L-tryptophan, 5-HTP, L-theanine, GABA, magnesium, and Sleepytime teas rather than prescribed drugs to help you sleep.

Chapter 7

PUTTING STRESS, ANXIETY, FEAR, AND WORRY TO BED

A S A PRACTICING medical doctor for more than twenty-five years, I have seen a dramatic rise in both depression and anxiety in my patients. The statistics on mental health disorders are absolutely staggering in the United States. It is estimated that in any given year 26.2 percent of adult Americans—about one in every four people—suffer from a diagnosable mental disorder.[1] This figure translates to approximately 57.7 million people.[2]

Americans are also typically stressed to the maximum—and the stress level is increasing. Today's newspapers and twenty-four-hour news networks often report news—such as threats of war and terrorism—that provoke people to become depressed and anxious.

And what many Americans are experiencing firsthand is even more stressful than what they see on the news. Due to the downward spiral in the economy, many Americans lost their jobs, lost their homes to foreclosure, or lost a large amount of their savings in the stock market. Many people who still have jobs are working longer and harder at the same jobs—some for less pay and with less employee benefits.

Then there is family stress—not having enough hours in the day to get everything done. Also, many families have been broken through divorce or blended together through remarriage, creating even more stress. Many teens are rebelling or abusing drugs. Even children worry about things they used to never have to worry about, such as gang violence, school shootings, and child abductions.

Situations like these can cause even the most optimistic of us to become stressed, anxious, worried, fearful, or a little down.

WIPING OUT WORRY

Every day I encounter patients in my office who tell me they are worried about a wide variety of things:

- "I'm afraid I'm going to lose my job."
- "I'm worried that I might have cancer."
- "I'm worried that I might develop heart disease or Alzheimer's disease."
- "I'm worried about my children."
- "I'm worried that I might lose my hair."
- "I'm worried that my wife might have an affair."
- "I'm worried that I won't be able to pay all my bills."

The list of things people worry about seems endless at times! We seem to be a nation of worriers.

I'm not talking now about the anxiety disorders that have been diagnosed in approximately nineteen million Americans.

These anxiety disorders include generalized anxiety disorder, post-traumatic stress disorder, obsessive-compulsive disorder, panic disorder, and phobias of many types. Rather, I'm talking about the tens of millions who suffer from mild anxiety that has not yet reached the level of a disorder. They have developed a habit of worrying.

Being a "worry wart" does not mean that a person is mentally ill. It just means that worry has become a mental habit. The habit can lead to a neurotransmitter imbalance in the brain, so in one sense, worry may lead to mental illness. In most cases people who worry do not need medication. They simply need to change their mental habits!

WORRY AND ANXIETY ARE UNHEALTHY

Anxiety is commonly referred to as the "common cold of mental illness." Worry and anxiety are virtually interchangeable terms. In fact, one dictionary defines *worry* as "to feel anxious." That same dictionary defines *anxiety* as "a concern that causes worry."

Both worry and anxiety are internal, unpleasant clusters of "nervous" or agitated thoughts and feelings that something unpleasant may happen or may already have happened. Worry and anxiety tend to be related to things we think about, imagine, or perceive. Worry and anxiety can be short term or long term—they can become almost a state of mind. Some people worry about everything!

The terms "anxiety attack" and "panic attack" have now been given to an intense bout of worry or anxiety in which the heart rate increases and a person may hyperventilate, sweat or tremble, feel weak, or have stomach or intestinal discomfort.

You Need New Software

Most of the thought patterns you have today have been learned from your parents or other figures of authority. When you were born, your mind was like a brand-new computer with brand-new software. Your thinking "powers up" your computer and launches the "operating software" that runs your life. Your parents or the people who raised you were the primary programmers of that operating software. If your parents programmed it with praise, contentment, gratitude, love, and joy, you are likely to go through life with these types of attitudes and expectations.

But if they programmed it with worry, you will be prone to worry; if they programmed it with fear, your automatic reaction is fear; if they programmed it with expecting the worst, you will expect the worst. Your parents may have programmed limitation into your thought patterns by telling you that you will never be smart enough, you will never make it, you will never be successful, or you are not talented enough.

My purpose is not to have you start blaming your parents—after all, their thought patterns were likely programmed by their parents, who were programmed by their parents, and so on. My goal is simply to help you understand where your thought patterns originated.

It actually all began when Adam and Even disobeyed God in the Garden of Eden. They allowed the virus of sin to infect the hardware of humanity, and from that point on, every heart and mind has been infected. We have been programmed with depraved thinking, negativity, hopelessness, anger, and insecurity.

When Christians are born again, we receive Christ's

forgiveness for our sins and invite Him into our hearts, but many Christians never purge the bad software from their minds even though the virus of sin has been removed. We need to learn to identify the feelings, thoughts, and beliefs that are distortional and replace them with the Word of God until God's thoughts and beliefs are automatic in our minds and in our hearts.

REPROGRAMMING YOUR DISTORTIONAL THOUGHTS

Think about our computer virus illustration for a moment. What happens when a virus gets into even the best computer and contaminates its software? At first, certain parts of the computer will not function properly, and it loses speed. Eventually the computer freezes and eventually may not run anymore.

So it is with your mind. Sinful viruses infect your life, contaminating your software with bitterness, unforgiveness, resentment, hatred, jealousy, anger, rage, and more. If allowed to spread throughout your system, they can affect your ability to function properly, just like a computer. Soon, not only are your mental health and emotional health affected, but also your physical health suffers too, leading to depression, anxiety, and a host of physical diseases.

The good news is that there are only ten major distortional beliefs that need to be reprogrammed. Let's take a look at them now.

1. All-or-nothing thinking

For this kind of person, there are no gray areas. Anything less than his standard of "perfect" is worthless.

Marty had this type of thinking. She was a high school senior assigned to write a term paper. She worked on the paper every night and weekend for two months, and when the paper was due, Marty didn't feel at all ready to turn it in. She feared receiving an F for not turning in a paper, however, so she hesitantly handed in the work she had done. She made an A- on the paper, but because she demanded perfection of herself, she saw an A- as a totally unacceptable grade. It might as well have been an F to her.

A healthy thinker recognizes that even in the best of circumstances, nothing or no one is perfect.

2. Overgeneralizations

A person who overgeneralizes thinks that if one thing goes wrong, nothing will ever go right for him ever.

Ed was an experienced civil engineer who had been with his last employer for more than twenty years. After his last employer filed for bankruptcy, he knew he would have to find another job that could offer the same pay scale, but he wondered who would hire an older, experienced engineer when they could hire a college graduate for less. After three interviews, a phone call, and two rejection letters, Ed concluded that third company would reject him, so he gave up any hope of finding another job.

If Ed were a healthy thinker, he would recognize that simply because company #3 has not replied, it is not a sign that he did not get the job. Instead he should remain positive, follow up the interview with a phone call thanking them for the interview, and wait for their reply.

3. A negative mental filter

This kind of distortional thinking causes a person to hear a half hour of praise after a job evaluation but leave the meeting depressed because of one area "needing improvement."

Anne was going to her high school prom. Her mother bought her a new dress and shoes and took her to have her hair professionally styled on the day of the prom. At the prom everyone complimented her on how beautiful she looked and how pretty her dress and hair were. One classmate who was jealous of Anne pointed out a run in her stockings. It was a very tiny run that was barely noticeable. Anne, however, felt mortified, as if every person in the room were aware of this flaw.

When Anne returned home that night and her mother asked about the prom, Anne focused so much on her embarrassment and her classmate's negative comment that Anne completely forgot about all the compliments she had received.

Choosing to focus only on the negative causes unnecessary stress. On the other hand, choosing to always focus only on the positive and not dealing with the negative is equally harmful and unrealistic. A person has to find the balance between the positive and negative situations in life.

4. Disqualifying the positive

Even more distortional is when a person takes a positive experience and turns it into a negative one. These kind of thinkers feel they are not worthy of any praise under any circumstance.

Harry was a faithful, hardworking salesman who had made his sales quota each of the last five years. Harry was promoted to sales director over the entire company, which was a great surprise to Harry. With the promotion came nearly a doubling of his salary. Rather than showing excitement about the possibility for this advancement, Harry immediately began to tell his supervisor that he didn't deserve the position. He pointed out several of his weaknesses and said that he thought a fellow worker named Steve was better qualified. Even though his supervisor pointed out several of his strengths, Harry discounted each of them. In the end, Harry sabotaged his own promotion.

Enjoy receiving compliments and praise, and use them to validate your self-esteem. There is nothing prideful about graciously accepting praise or a compliment when rightfully given. Not only will this reduce stress, but it will also add richness to your life.

5. Jumping to conclusions

People who jump to conclusions predict the worst possible outcome or circumstance without having any, or all, the facts to support their conclusions.

One day Jeanette overhears her boss speaking with someone about a job description very similar to her own. Immediately Jeanette thought, "He's not happy with my work, and he's going to replace me with this person. What am I going to do if I get fired?" Her boss notifies her that he has something to tell her later in the day. All afternoon her stomach is in knots. Trying to concentrate on her work is impossible. It is almost time for Jeanette to go home, when a young woman walks in the door and her boss says, "Jeanette, I'd like for you to meet my niece. She was just hired as a receptionist at our other office. We are so pleased with your work that I want you to train her." Jeanette jumped to the conclusion that she was losing her job to another person, which was not the case at all.

Instead of getting stressed out about the thought of losing her job, Jeanette should have waited until her boss spoke with her before drawing a conclusion about the situation.

6. Magnification or minimization

Dr. David Burns, author of *Feeling Good: The New Mood Therapy*, refers to magnification also as *catastrophizing*. A person who "awful-izes" the possibility of a disaster tends to magnify, or blow out of proportion, the importance of circumstances or a situation. A simple mishap, however small, is regarded as a monumental disaster. Some people also call this "Murphy's Law" mentality: "If anything can go wrong, it will go wrong, and it will be worse because that's just my luck."

Beth realized her boss was overwhelmed and volunteered to help prepare a report for the stockholder's meeting. The day after the meeting, her boss came in very grumpy. He complained about a few things, and Beth became flustered. She thought, "What made me think I could prepare that report? Maybe there was a spelling error. I feel terrible!" She began visualizing her boss giving the report and becoming embarrassed because of her imaginary mistakes. Later that day her boss apologized for his behavior. He explained that he hadn't slept well the night before because he had a painful backache. He thanked Beth for being so understanding and for the fine job she did composing the report.

The person who magnifies perceived weaknesses also tends to minimize his personal success as inconsequential. In this example Beth underestimated her ability to put together a well-written report.

The healthy thinker sees life as a sequence of events, all of which are factored into an overall track record. No single event is perceived as being overly important or of no consequence.

7. Emotional reasoning

This person allows the truth to be based upon his feelings. If he feels incompetent, then he thinks he must be doing a lousy job.

Terry had just graduated from college and had accepted a position for a large company selling life insurance. He was very excited about the possibility of making a lot of money. However, after the first week, he had been turned down by every prospect. He felt rejected, depressed, and worthless. He took it personally that people were rejecting him instead of realizing that they were rejecting the life insurance. He allowed his feelings and emotions to affect his job, and he eventually quit.

The healthy thinker separates his emotions from his overall self-worth.

8. "Should" statements—fixed-rule thinking

This person is a "should," "must," or "ought to" person. He confines people and events to his rules and fails to realize the fact that he can't force anyone to adhere to them. The more rigid the rules, the greater the person's disappointment. That disappointment usually plays out as worry, depression, frustration, irritation, or guilt.

Mr. Smith, CEO of XYZ Company, is attending an industry convention. He has Susan, his executive assistant, make hotel reservations months in advance at the host hotel. The day before he is scheduled to check in to the hotel, he has Susan call to confirm.

She reports back that the hotel could not find his reservation, even though Susan has a confirmation number. Now there is no room available because they are booked solid due to the convention. Mr. Smith blows up at Susan, blaming her for the lost reservation. After all, "she should've made sure his reservation was secure." The person with fixed-rule thinking tends to live in "should" statements. People should do certain things, society should act a particular way, or a situation should turn out in an expected fashion.

The healthy thinker knows that the only "should" statement a person should make is one in the form of a question: "How should I approach this situation now and in the future?"

9. Labeling and mislabeling

A person who attaches a negative label to himself or someone else tends to do so because of his own low self-esteem.

Many children, unfortunately, are called names such as *stupid*, *lazy*, or *no good*. Then those children call other people by these names or may call themselves by these names, at least in their own minds. If a person labels himself as stupid or lazy long enough, eventually he will live up to that label. It becomes a self-fulfilling prophecy.

Early in his childhood Johnny had been diagnosed with attention deficit hyperactivity disorder (ADHD). He frequently fought with other children and would end up in the principal's office. He had difficulty staying quiet in class and wouldn't do his homework. He ended up failing two grades and, as a result, was much bigger than the other kids in his class.

When Johnny became a teenager, he began using drugs and alcohol, and eventually he became a drug dealer. He covered his body with tattoos and had piercings in his ears, tongue, lip, eyebrow, and chin. He was big, strong, and scary-looking—highly intimidating to other teenagers. Those who had picked on him and called him names when he was younger were now frequently threatened with bodily harm if they didn't buy drugs from him.

As a result, a number of his schoolmates were hooked on drugs and dependent on him to supply them. Johnny had no respect whatsoever for those to whom he sold drugs. His "names" for them were often spoken in derision and with expletives.

Johnny was a victim of labeling and name-calling, but he also became a person who labeled and called others names. The cycle of name-calling is often a downward one.

Remember that God has called you precious and beloved, and you are His child.

10. Personalization

This kind of thinking shifts the blame of an outcome on self. Unfortunately in our society, many children who come from dysfunctional homes become trapped in this kind of thinking: "Daddy left Mommy because I was bad."

After Amy's father died, her mother, Nancy, was left with the financial burden of a home and raising Amy alone. Amy's mother began drinking to numb her emotional pain and drown her problems. Amy blames herself for her mother's alcohol addiction and feels that if she were not in the house, then her mother would be free to sell the house and go on with her life. Rather than feel guilty, Amy needs to realize that her mother is an adult who needs help and needs to learn to cope with life's situations.

Free yourself of stress and guilt by realizing that you are not responsible for another person's actions or decisions. In the case of a child, the child needs to be reassured that he did nothing wrong and that his dad's decision to leave was not his fault.

For more information on distortional thinking, read my book *Deadly Emotions*.

ANSWERING THE QUESTION: WHO OWES WHOM?

Many of these distortional thoughts are rooted in a general overriding belief that life owes a person something. There is nothing written in the cosmos or the Word of God that declares this to be true. Life owes you nothing; you owe life something!

People who think life owes them something are always blaming others for their own failures, shortcomings, and even their own stress! How often do we hear statements like these: "My boss makes me nervous." "My husband frustrates me." "My children annoy me." "My neighbors stress me out." Many things don't happen to us intentionally; things happen as part of the overall "life experience."

Sadly, most stressed-out people don't realize that a very high percentage of their stress is the result of distortional thinking. This is especially true if they are blaming others for their stress. Such a person rarely looks in the mirror and says, "I'm causing these stressful feelings in my life."

Putting Your Thoughts on Trial

Most of these thoughts are under the radar because you have been practicing them so much that they have become mind-sets. You may fly off the handle or become anxious over a minor event or circumstance without even thinking about it, or you feel stress, depression, or anxiety, and you don't even realize that you don't have to react this way.

In order to recognize these patterns, you must first tune in to your feelings and take inventory of what you are thinking. By monitoring your feelings you will eventually be able to figure out which thoughts and beliefs triggered your anxiety. I call these "thought triggers." The thought triggers are almost always one of these ten distortional thought patterns that have become ingrained in your thinking similar to a computer virus. The first step in breaking this stronghold is to identify these triggers.

It is also helpful to journal your thoughts, to write down exactly what is going through your mind when you are feeling depressed or anxious. (Remember, depressed or anxious feelings mean that you are usually thinking a distortional thought pattern or reliving or rehashing a traumatic event.)

Next, compare the thoughts you've written down in your journal to the list of ten distortional thought patterns. Then begin confessing the positive confessions from God's Word that correspond to the negative thoughts you've identified in your journal.

I call this "taking your distortional thought patterns to court." You see, most people believe that these patterns are true since they have been thinking this way all of their lives. However, you need to put these thought patterns and assumptions on trial, convict them, imprison them, and then reprogram them with God's Word. Unfortunately most Christians have not done this, and that is why just as many Christians have depression and anxiety as non-Christians.

I also recommend that you seek the advice of a good cognitive-behavioral therapist to ensure that you identify and change these distortional thought patterns. I commonly refer my patients to this kind of therapist and find that people with depression as well as all types of anxiety disorders will usually benefit significantly from cognitive-behavioral therapy.

As a physician, I am trained to carefully examine my patients and prescribe any medicines or lifestyle changes that may be necessary. I have found that my most powerful prescription for healthy living can't be found in a bottle or at a pharmacist's counter. It has one exclusive source, and it is freely available to everyone. I am talking about the Word of God, of course. Joy and peace can come to even the most troubled minds when people discover new ways of looking at life based upon the truth of God's wonderful Word.

z Building Blocks to a Better z Night's Sleep

- A lot of problems in our world and our individual lifestyle choices can lead to stress, anxiety, fear, and worry—but this is not how God designed you to live. It's time to put them to bed!

- Most of our worries, stresses, and fears can be eliminated through a reprogramming of our distortional thoughts. Put your distortional thoughts on trial to discover they don't hold weight.

Chapter 8

FIND YOUR REST IN GOD

YOU MIGHT BE surprised to hear this, but the amount of stress and turmoil you experience in your daily life does not truly indicate how well you will sleep. One person's life can be full of stress-producing events and situations, and yet this person will be at rest. Another individual's life can be comparatively free of stress, and yet this individual might be filled with tension, turmoil, panic, and distress. The difference between the two individuals is not how much stress they encounter, but rather whether or not they are abiding in the vine.

Let me explain. The Bible says, "Abide in Me, and I in you. As the branch cannot bear fruit of itself, unless it abides in the vine, neither can you, unless you abide in Me. I am the vine, you are the branches. He who abides in Me, and I in him, bears much fruit; for without Me you can do nothing" (John 15:4–5).

Experiencing a restful life comes from abiding in Christ. This simply means giving Him all of your anxiety, care, and concern and receiving from Him His wisdom, peace, power, and love. This wonderful spiritual exchange produces blessed rest in God.

So you can see that what really matters is not the amount of stress or activity in your life but how you actually perceive what's happening and how you react to it. If you react with worry, anger, rage, fear, resentment, or any other deadly emotion, you're liable to lose a lot of sleep and peace. But if you react to the stress in your life with faith, trust, peace, and reassurance that God is in control, you'll continue to sleep like a baby through every ripple and wave you encounter.

Still, appearances can be deceiving. Sometimes a person who appears calm outwardly can be steaming internally. But it's often difficult to mask your emotions at 2:00 a.m. when you are lying awake staring at the ceiling, replaying the day or planning tomorrow. So if you are struggling to get a good night's sleep, your reactions to stress and other deadly emotions may be a key factor.

Therefore, be sure that you're abiding in the vine. Let's examine some ways you can do this.

Start With Scripture

Psalm 127:2 says, "It is vain for you to rise up early, to sit up late, to eat the bread of sorrows; for so He gives His beloved sleep." The Bible actually promises us a good night's sleep, but we have to do our part in order to obtain it. We unknowingly eat the bread of sorrows by rehashing the stresses and worries of the day and being more concerned about things for tomorrow. We lie in bed at night trying to figure things out. That is vain!

Instead, we need to meditate on God's Word and not on our problems and stresses. As we meditate on God's Word, our problems go. But as we meditate on the problem, our problems grow, and as a result, our sleep is destroyed. Isaiah

26:3 says, "You will keep him in perfect peace, whose mind is stayed on You." In other words, as we keep our minds on God's Word and not our problems, we will enter into peace.

Our minds must be renewed, just as Romans 12:1–2 says, so that they will be on the side of the Spirit, who is perfect. This renewing of the mind occurs as our thoughts are filled with the powerful, living Word of God. But if our minds are always thinking upon negatives, such as what makes us worry or angry, what we don't have that we want, who has hurt us or caused us harm, and what we dislike, then our minds and thoughts are carnal or inspired by our lower nature. When we fill our minds with God's words and thoughts through the Bible and prayer, we feed and strengthen our spirit man, which was designed to serve God.

The Obedience of Rest

One of the best ways to wind down is to understand and follow God's law of rest. Let's take a look at this incredible law. The Word of God says, "And six years thou shalt sow thy land, and shalt gather the fruits thereof: but the seventh year thou shalt let it rest and lie still. . . . Six days thou shalt do thy work, and on the seventh day thou shalt rest" (Exod. 23:10–12, KJV).

You can find this same powerful spiritual principle in Exodus 31:15: "Six days may work be done; but in the seventh is the sabbath of rest, holy to the Lord: whosoever doeth any work in the sabbath day, he shall surely be put to death" (KJV). The next verse goes on to say that this was a perpetual covenant—which means that this principle of Sabbath rest never ends. And verse 17 says, "It is a sign between me and the children of Israel *for ever*: for in six days the Lord made heaven and earth, and on the seventh day he rested, and was refreshed" (KJV, emphasis added).

Today we are not under law, but we live under the grace of God that was purchased for us by Christ Jesus. Nevertheless, rest remains a spiritual principle that we cannot disregard without suffering heavy consequences in terms of our health and well-being.

Although we don't honor the Sabbath by strictly forbidding work on Sundays, we enter into a rest when we learn to depend upon God for everything in our lives. The New Testament talks about this rest when it says, "So there remains a Sabbath rest for the people of God" (Heb. 4:9, NAS).

So you can see that rest remains a very present and powerful spiritual principle that God gave to strengthen our bodies and minds and renew our health and spirits. By honoring the Sabbath rest of God, we rest our bodies and our minds. We refuse to carry around the weight of the daily tension, anxiety, fear, and stress of the world. Instead, we let God carry it for us. In doing so, we enter God's rest.

The powerful spiritual principle of God's rest allows our minds and bodies to heal from the effects of stress. Jesus says, "Come to Me, all you who labor and are heavy laden, and I will give you rest" (Matt. 11:28). God's rest is a vital key factor in living in God's divine health for your body, mind, and soul.

We need to enter into the sleep and rest of Jesus. In Matthew 8 Jesus and His disciples got in a boat, and suddenly a great tempest, or storm, arose on the sea. The wind was probably howling and the boat was rocking violently. The Bible says in verse 24 that the boat was covered with waves, or in other words, it was about to sink. But in spite of the violent rocking of the boat, the howling winds, and the waves crashing over the boat, Jesus was sound asleep. No doubt He was in stage four sleep, which is the deepest stage of sleep.

But then His disciples came and woke Him up and said to Him, "Lord, save us! We are perishing!" He then asked them, "Why are you fearful, O you of little faith?" He then got up and rebuked the winds and the sea, and there was a great calm. The key here is that we too can enter into His rest and sweet sleep just like Jesus if we abide in Him and He abides in us.

A LOVING LIFE

First Corinthians 13:8 says, "Love never fails." Are you in a political battle at work? Do you have strife in your family? Have you been hurt by your spouse? Love truly never fails—and it will not fail you! Can you imagine, there is only one thing the Bible tells us will never fail us, and that is practicing the love walk. We need to practice all the characteristics of love in 1 Corinthians 13:4–7. I recommend reading this passage aloud and inserting yourself in place of *love* in these verses:

> Love is patient and kind. [I am patient and kind.] Love is not jealous or boastful or proud or rude. [I am not jealous or boastful or proud or rude.] It does not demand its own way. [I do not demand my own way.] It is not irritable, and it keeps no record of being wronged. [I am not irritable, and I keep no record of being wronged.] It does not rejoice about injustice but rejoices whenever the truth wins out. [I do not rejoice about injustice but rejoice whenever the truth wins out.] Love never gives up, never loses faith, is always

hopeful, and endures through every circumstance. [I never give up, never lose faith, am always hopeful, and endure through every circumstance.]

1 CORINTHIANS 13:4–7, NLT

Notice that love keeps no record of wrongs. In other words, forgiveness is part of love. Throw away the record-keeping book and forgive everyone who has wronged you. As Christians there is only one commandment we have, and it is the love commandment. (See John 13:34.)

Fear rules the lives of many people, but the Bible says, "Perfect love casts out fear" (1 John 4:18). You can live free from fear as you increasingly understand the power of God's love for you. Mahatma Gandhi said that the whole world would accept the Christ of Christians if the Christians would only act like Christ.

Build and maintain the ties of relationships. Relationships with those who love you are gifts from God. Never take them for granted!

THE PURSUIT OF HAPPINESS

According to Rich Bayer, PhD, CEO of Upper Bay Counseling and Support Services, Inc., happy people have more social contact and better social relations than their unhappy counterparts. Studies of positive people show that they rate high on having good relationships with themselves and with others. Their love for life is better as well. Happy people tend to be kinder to others and to express empathy more easily.

Of course, happy people are not luckier than other people. They experience their share of tragedy and hardship, but studies show that they do a better job of reframing what happens to them.[1] They remember the good events in their lives more readily, and when bad things happen, they believe things will eventually be all right. They have hope.

Happiness is one of the keys to a long, satisfying life. Studies also show that happy people have fewer health problems.[2] Research among older people indicates that folks with positive emotions outlive their sour counterparts. Happy people were shown to be half as likely to become disabled as sad people in the same age bracket. And happy people have a higher pain threshold than those who are sad.[3]

WHAT WILL YOU CHOOSE?

Worry and fear are the opposite of faith and peace. We are told in the Bible to cast all our care upon the Lord. (See 1 Peter 5:7.) God did not say *some* of your cares—He said *all*.

Jesus had this to say about worry:

> Therefore do not worry, saying, "What shall we eat?" or "What shall we drink?" or "What shall we wear?" For after all these things the Gentiles seek. For your heavenly Father knows that you need all these things. But seek first the kingdom of God and His righteousness, and all these things shall be added to you. Therefore do not worry about tomorrow, for tomorrow will worry about its own things. Sufficient for the day is its own trouble.
>
> —MATTHEW 6:31–34

Faith is simply trusting God to do what He has promised to do in the Bible. It means trusting Him to forgive you because He said He would forgive you if you confessed your sins to Him and asked Him to forgive you. (See 1 John 1:9.) It means trusting Him to care for you because He says He cares for you. (See 1 Peter 5:7.) It means trusting Him to love you because He says He loves you. (See 1 John 4:19.)

How do we acquire faith? The Bible tells us that we each have already been given a measure of faith (Rom. 12:3). The challenge before us is to grow in our faith. We do this by hearing the Word of God (Rom. 10:17). This does not simply mean we listen to sermons and tapes of good Bible preaching and teaching. It means that we study and meditate on God's Word. As part of studying and meditating, we are wise to read God's Word aloud and to memorize Scripture so we can meditate on God's Word any place and any time.

When we read the Bible aloud to ourselves, we are "hearing" the Word of God. When we repeat God's Word aloud to ourselves in the process of memorizing it, we are "hearing" the Word of God. When we recite God's Word from memory to ourselves, we are "hearing" the Word of God. The two ears closest to your mouth when you speak are likely to be your ears! The Bible tells us, "You will keep him in perfect peace, whose mind is stayed on You" (Isa. 26:3). What will you choose to hear?

PRACTICING MINDFULNESS

The concept of mindfulness, studied and explained best by Herbert Benson, MD, is the practice of learning to pay attention to what is happening to you from moment to moment. To be mindful, according to Benson, you must slow down, do one activity at a time, and bring your full awareness to both the activity at hand and to your inner experience of it.[4] Mindfulness provides a potentially powerful antidote to the common causes of daily stress.

Choose Your Company Wisely

DR. COLBERT APPROVED

Make a conscious decision to limit the amount of time you spend with negative, pessimistic people. They not only will sabotage your goals, but they will also drain energy from you. I call these people "energy vampires" or "energy leeches" because no matter what you do, they seem to make you "tired" by their endless whining, complaining, and bickering. Avoid this frustration by avoiding or limiting your time spent with such people.

Benson's definition of mindfulness reminds me of the words of Jesus: "Therefore do not worry about tomorrow, for tomorrow will worry about its own things. Sufficient for the day is its own trouble" (Matt. 6:34). Jesus taught us to be mindful of the present, not of the future. The apostle Paul likewise taught us to forget "those things which are behind," meaning the past (Phil. 3:13). Mindfulness means letting go of any thought that is unrelated to the present moment and finding something to enjoy in the present moment.

But most people do not live in the present moment. They are wishing for a different moment—either past or future. They go through the motions required to function in the present moment, but they are thinking things like "I'll be happy when..."

153

- "I get a bigger home."

- "I get that promotion."

- "My kids are out of school."

- "I pay off these bills."

- "I get a new car."

- "I lose twenty pounds."

Mindfulness works differently. It trains your mind to let go of any thought that is unrelated to the present moment and to find something to enjoy in the present—continually. When you walk or drive, pay attention to the beautiful scenery, the chirping of the birds and crickets, and the feel of the warm sunshine or the chill in the air. Focus on the way your body feels as you go through routine motions of driving, opening the door, walking to your destination. During work breaks and in the evening refuse to think about goals, projects, or tasks that are not part of the present moment. If a stressful thought comes to mind, choose to move on to a thought that is related to what you are presently seeing, hearing, smelling, or feeling.

If you have to stop at a red light while driving to work, don't get frustrated, but consider it a welcome opportunity to be thankful for your car, your job, your boss, and so on. The majority of people in third world countries would love to have your car, your job, and your boss. Quit complaining about what you don't have, and start practicing gratitude for what you do have. You can practice gratitude by enjoying the music, the sights around you, the fact that you have air conditioning or heating for your car or house, and the fact that you have a car and are well enough to drive.

As you practice mindfulness, your muscles will relax, your body unwinds, and your stress is relieved. I encourage my patients to take a drive in the country, take a walk, play with children or grandchildren, smell the flowers, or go to the zoo and look at the animals. This teaches them to get absorbed in the present moment so their minds can de-stress naturally.

My favorite way to practice mindfulness is taking my grandson Braden to the park. He is so excited and runs to the slide and slides down and then climbs back up the slide again. He then loves to stop and pick up wood chips on the ground and then stick them in any tiny little hole he finds, which is usually in the playground equipment. One day he sat for an hour near the top of the slide simply breaking off little twigs and sticking them through the small holes in the flooring of the playground equipment. He also loves to run and have me chase him, saying, "Papa, get me!" He gets so tickled that he falls to the ground. He then looks up in the sky and loves to see airplanes. But his favorite sight is seeing the moon every night. In watching Braden, I enjoy practicing mindfulness.

To have complete mental and physical health, mindfulness must become a way of life, a continual pattern for practicing relaxation during your day. Make mindfulness a habit by practicing it daily.

THE MEDICINE OF LAUGHTER

The Bible says, "A merry heart does good, like medicine" (Prov. 17:22). If you are stressed out, why not take a prescription for laughter? When you're down or stressed, pick up a wholesome, funny video and watch it. A good, strong twenty-second belly laugh is equivalent to three minutes on a rowing machine, according to one study.[5] Laughter releases tension, anxiety, anger, fear, shame, and guilt, and it can transform your attitude and outlook.

When people come into my office to be treated or placed on a nutritional program, I often ask them, "How often do you laugh?" You should see the looks they give me. A common response in cancer patients is, "I never laugh." I can tell they're thinking, "I have cancer, Dr. Colbert. What is there to laugh about?"

One of the most unusual prescriptions I give to many of my patients is to have at least ten belly laughs a day, with each belly laugh lasting at least twenty seconds. True laughing offers one of the most powerful and natural healing methods without any side effects. Laughter lowers the stress hormones cortisol and epinephrine. It increases feel-good hormones. It keeps you squarely in the present moment practicing mindfulness. It helps you to reframe and feel thankful and helps you to see negative events in a more positive light. There's not a single bad thing laughter will do for your body and mind.

A FITTING WORD

You may not want to admit it, but you probably talk to yourself from time to time. Don't worry; it is very normal. In fact, the most important conversations that we have are those we have with ourselves! Unfortunately we tend to have mostly negative conversations with ourselves. This is bound to have a poor outcome, as it means our minds are constantly barraged by nagging negative thoughts that beat us down a little lower each day. Who can thrive in such an environment?

Dr. Colbert APPROVED

Ten Benefits of Laughter

- It relieves stress and tension, decreases stress hormones, and helps you relax.
- It improves sleep.
- It helps balance neurotransmitters, helping to relieve anxiety and depression.
- It relieves pain.
- It strengthens relationships.
- It improves the immune system.
- It's like internal jogging. One belly laugh (about twenty seconds of "guffawing") is equivalent to exercising three minutes on a rowing machine.[6]
- It may help to prevent heart attack. Research shows that people with heart disease are 40 percent less likely to laugh in various situations.[7]
- It's good for the brain and can increase problem solving and creativity.
- It increases longevity. Bob Hope and George Burns both lived to be one hundred years of age.

I have seen fathers at Little League baseball games constantly criticizing their children, calling them stupid, dumb, pitiful—saying that they can't do anything right. I have seen the poor children standing in the outfield or slumped over sitting on the bench with dejected, depressed looks on their little faces. Unfortunately some of these children who have been told that they are losers, that they are dumb, stupid, and can never do anything right, grow up to believe those words. They become depressed, unmotivated, and unsuccessful people.

If a person feeds on negative thoughts throughout the day, every task or every trial that comes his way will be approached from a defeated attitude before he even undertakes it. However, we have the ability, through the Word of God, to speak God's Word throughout the day and rewire these negative thoughts into positive thoughts, which will then bring healing and health to the body and the mind.

THOUGHTS OF JOY

If you intend to live at peace, it is important for you to train your mind to think positive thoughts rather than dwelling on the negative. When a negative thought pops into your mind, it is important to cast down that thought and to speak out the solution, which is the Word of God. That is why memorizing and quoting scriptures is so important. Biblical, positive thoughts lead to winning attitudes.

An attitude is a choice. You can choose to have a negative attitude, or you can choose to have a positive attitude. You can choose to be angry, bitter, resentful, unforgiving, fearful, or ashamed. These negative attitudes eventually affect your health and allow diseases to take root in your body.

LET IT GO

When Paul and Silas were placed in prison, they prayed and sang praises (Acts 16:23–25). Paul had a choice. He could have had a negative attitude and become angry, resentful, and bitter. Instead, he chose to rejoice and sing praises. He chose the healthy attitude. He decided to "always be joyful" (1 Thess. 5:16, NLT).

When an individual wrongs you, it is very easy to hold bitterness, resentment, anger, and unforgiveness. However, this works against your body and will actually cause disease to set in. Resentment and unforgiveness are commonly associated with fibromyalgia and arthritis, and fear is commonly associated with cancer. Anxiety is commonly associated with ulcers, and anger is commonly associated with heart disease. These are deadly emotions. If they are not taken out of us through the Word of God or with the help of a trained professional, they can eventually lead to disease. It is far better for your body—for both your mental and physical health—to forgive the person and release these deadly emotions before they take root in your mind, emotions, and body.

The Bible says it plainly: "Do not let the sun go down on your wrath" (Eph. 4:26). This, I believe, is one of the most important keys in preventing these deadly emotions from locking onto our minds, emotions, and bodies and eventually killing us.

Paul decided to forget those things that were behind him and to press forward to the prize of the mark of the high calling in Christ Jesus. (See Philippians 3:14.) Choose the right attitude as soon as you wake up in the morning. When someone wrongs you, forgive that person immediately. Do not focus on the wrong.

WHAT IF YOU HAD JUST SIX MORE MONTHS?

I have treated a lot of patients with only six months or less to live. Many of these individuals have given up most of their distortional thought patterns, forgiven people whom they were angry with, and decided to live the remainder of their life in peace. It is truly incredible what comes into focus when you are facing the end of your life.

And so I like to invite my other patients—the ones seeing me for other ailments but who aren't living in dire straits—to try out what I call the "six-months-to-live test." The philosophy is very similar to the Tim McGraw song "Live Like You Were Dying." It's a chance to ask the question, "If I were given six months to live, what would I change?" It's a chance to find out what's most important—and then to live life accordingly.

I have helped many of these patients forgive, accept, and love themselves. Most of these patients were tired of the world's treadmill of work, work, work. Instead of human beings, many had become "human doings." Many seemed almost relieved to be able to have an excuse to get off the world's treadmill.

With this test many people are able to reframe their thought patterns and see people, circumstances, and even their disease from a different perspective. They give up distortional thought patterns, hurts, bitterness, depression, and anxiety, and they forgive themselves and others and accept and love themselves and others. Will you be among those who thrive in the face of such an invitation?

A GRATEFUL LIFE

One of the most powerful ways to lean into a life of rest is simply to practice gratitude. In the past few years there has been considerable research on living with a mind-set of gratitude. Researchers have found that gratitude helps you create a higher income, create superior work outcomes, experience a longer and better marriage, have more friends, have stronger social supports, have more energy, enjoy better overall physical health, develop a stronger immune system, have better cardiovascular health, lower your stress levels, and enjoy a longer life (up to ten years longer in one study).[8]

Research also proves that expressing gratitude makes everyone happier. Most people wrongly believe that happiness comes from what we buy, what we achieve, or where we go on vacation. That is simply not true; true happiness and joy come from within, and gratitude is a great way to gain access to this joy. Grateful people also sleep better, take better care of themselves, eat a healthier diet, exercise more regularly, and have less depression and anxiety and more enthusiasm and optimism.

I love this quote from Melody Beattie:

> Gratitude unlocks the fullness of life. It turns what we have into enough, and more. It turns denial into acceptance, chaos to order, confusion to clarity. It can turn a meal into a feast, a house into a home, and a stranger into a friend. Gratitude makes sense of our past, brings peace for today, and creates a vision for tomorrow.[9]

One of the best examples of gratitude is the story of the ten lepers in Luke chapter 17. During the days of Jesus the disease of leprosy was worse than AIDS. It usually started with disfiguring sores on the skin before advancing to nerve damage, fingers and toes falling off, and progressive disfigurement. It was also a very painful disease and, because there was no cure at that time, was actually a death sentence.

Once a person was identified as a leper, he or she was cast out of the city to live in a poor leper colony. A strict law stated that people could not even get within fifty yards of a leper because lepers were considered "unclean."

It was very rare to be healed of leprosy, but it did happen on rare occasions. To be allowed to leave the leper colony, a person was required to be examined by the priest and declared clean.

In Luke 17 Jesus looked at the ten lepers and said, "Go show yourselves to the priest." On their way to the priest they looked down and saw that their skin blotches were entirely gone and their leprosy was healed.

One of the lepers, a Samaritan, said, "Wait, I want to go back and thank Jesus." The other nine lepers were Jewish, but this one Samaritan leper (Samaritans were typically despised and treated as second-class citizens by most Jews) returned and threw himself down at Jesus's feet and thanked Him. Jesus then told the one leper to arise and go his way and that his faith had made him whole. Realize that *whole* means, according to Bible scholars, that missing body parts were restored. Why did Jesus do this? Because of the man's gratitude.

As in the case of the lepers, I believe that only about 10 percent (or less) of Christians practice gratitude on a regular basis. Therefore, there are just as many Christians suffering from a lack of joy and contentment in life as the rest of the world. Think that over: 90 percent of Christians never stop and thank God for all their blessings

It's time to stop complaining about what you do not have and start thanking God for what you do have. I often recommend that my patients make a gratitude journal. It can be a fancy journal you purchase from the store or a simple three-ring binder or spiral notebook.

In this journal you will want to write something you are thankful for each and every day. Be sure to include various body parts and functions, such as your vision; hearing; the ability to taste, smell, and touch; the ability to walk and to use fingers, arms, legs, toes, back, and neck. Be grateful for every aspect of your health.

Also in your gratitude journal should be a list of family and friends, your spouse, and other people God has brought into your life. Don't forget to be grateful for a hot shower, toilet, bed, refrigerator, stove, dishwasher, car, home, air conditioning, sufficient food, clothing, furniture, and so on.

Our thoughts lead to the words we say, and our words lead to our attitudes. We need to practice an attitude of gratitude. It is critically important to guard our thoughts and to quote the Word of God aloud throughout the day in order to produce godly attitudes within us. Nutrition, exercise, and adequate sleep are all important. However, our thoughts, beliefs, words, and attitudes will determine if we succeed or if we fail; they determine where we spend our eternity as well.

CONFESSIONS, AFFIRMATIONS, PRAYERS, AND SCRIPTURES FOR RESTING IN GOD

We've considered multiple ways to abide in the vine and find rest in this chapter. But what it ultimately boils down to is finding our rest in God. It's about keeping our minds stayed on God. It's about finding life in the Scriptures. It's about keeping attuned to God in prayer. It's about believing all the goodness God speaks over us.

In this section you'll find a ready arsenal of prayers, confessions, affirmations, and scriptures to keep you leaning into God, who is your ultimate sourse of rest.

CONFESSIONS FOR SLEEP

Scripture	My Confession
"I will both lie down in peace, and sleep; for You alone, O Lord, make me dwell in safety" (Ps. 4:8).	The Lord is watching over me and promises me peace, safety, and a good night's sleep. I receive peaceful sleep by faith.
"It is vain for you to rise up early, to sit up late, to eat the bread of sorrows; for so He gives His beloved sleep" (Ps. 127:2).	I am God's loved one, and He promises me rest. Thank You, Lord, for rest and sweet sleep as part of my inheritance and a free gift. I receive deep sleep by faith.
"You can go to bed without fear; you will lie down and sleep soundly" (Prov. 3:24, NLT).	I will not fear when I lie down because the peace of God rests on me. When I lie down, I will fall asleep, and my sleep will be peaceful, deep, and refreshing just like the sleep of Jesus.
"You will keep him in perfect peace, whose mind is stayed on You, because he trusts in You" (Isa. 26:3).	I have perfect peace because my mind is focused on Jesus and not on my problems.
"Then Jesus said, 'Come to me, all of you who are weary and carry heavy burdens, and I will give you rest'" (Matt. 11:28, NLT).	I give all my burdens to Jesus, and I enter into His rest. I have the peace of God and am able to sleep soundly.
"[Jesus said,] 'Peace I leave with you, My peace I give to you; not as the world gives do I give to you. Let not your heart be troubled, neither let it be afraid'" (John 14:27).	I receive the peace of God, the same peace that Jesus had by faith. That was the peace that enabled Him to be in a deep sleep in the midst of a bad storm at sea. His peace rests on me.

Scripture	My Confession
"Casting down arguments and every high thing that exalts itself against the knowledge of God, bringing every thought into captivity to the obedience of Christ" (2 Cor. 10:5).	I cast every worrisome thought and all other bothersome thoughts out of my mind, and I choose to focus on the name of Jesus. I slowly inhale and exhale as I think the name of Jesus, and I do not allow any other thoughts into my mind.
"Be anxious for nothing, but in everything by prayer and supplication, with thanksgiving, let your requests be made known to God; and the peace of God, which surpasses all understanding, will guard your hearts and minds through Christ Jesus" (Phil. 4:6–7).	The peace of God guards my heart and my mind. All thoughts contrary to God's Word are cast out of my mind by faith. Tormenting thoughts must leave, and I refuse to rehash those thoughts. I refuse to be anxious.
"For God has not given [me] a spirit of fear, but of power and of love and of a sound mind" (2 Tim. 1:7).	By faith I have a sound mind. No fear, anxiety, depression, insomnia, or worrisome thoughts can stay because God's Word says I have a sound mind.
"For only we who believe can enter his rest" (Heb. 4:3, NLT).	I believe and have entered into God's rest and peace.

Positive affirmations

I am beautiful, capable, and lovable. I am valuable. I have complete faith and trust in Jesus Christ. All of my needs are met. God shall supply all of my needs according to His riches and glory in Christ Jesus. I love myself unconditionally and nurture myself in every way. I trust my conscience, which is led by the Holy Spirit. I follow my conscience and choose to walk in the Spirit and not in the flesh.

I am a beautiful child of God. I am filled with love. I love people and radiate love, warmth, and friendship to all. I am healed of all my childhood wounds, and I am moving toward greater peace and happiness every day. I hold no account of wrong done to me.

I am diligent, faithful, and have a spirit of excellence. Whatever I put my hand to will prosper. I am the head and not the tail. God always causes me to triumph. I am unique and the apple of God's eye. The Greater One, Jesus, lives in me. I can be intimate with myself and others. I can love myself, and I can love others. I choose to love everyone with whom I come in contact. Love is patient; therefore, I am patient. Love is kind; therefore, I am kind. Love does not envy; therefore, I am content. Love does not exalt itself and is not proud; therefore, I am meek and humble. Love is not rude; therefore, I am courteous. Love is not selfish; therefore, I am giving. Love is not provoked; therefore, I am forgiving. Love thinks no evil. My thoughts are true, honest, just, pure, loving, and of good report. Love does not rejoice in iniquity but rejoices in the truth; therefore, I rejoice in the truth. Love bears all things, believes all things in God's Word, hopes all things, and endures all things. Love never fails; therefore, I will not fail.

Everything that happens to me I create consciously or unconsciously. I have made a decision not to judge anyone, including myself. Jesus said, "Judge not, and ye shall not be judged. Condemn not, and ye shall not be condemned. Forgive, and ye shall be forgiven" (Luke 6:37, kjv). I choose to forgive, and I will be forgiven. I choose to forgive everyone from whom I feel less than unconditional love. I choose to walk in unconditional love toward all men. I choose to see the best in everyone. I am open to new beliefs. I accept and love my parents.

I create my own happiness. I am appreciated, and I appreciate others. I make decisions with confidence. I let go of things I cannot control. I have the courage to change the things I should change. I have the serenity to accept the things I cannot change, and I have the wisdom to know the difference. I allow myself to play and have fun. I have no need to control people or situations. I release all need to control. I am controlled by the Holy Spirit.

All my needs, desires, and goals are met. Whatever I can conceive and believe, I can achieve. All things are possible to me because I believe. My capabilities and potential are unlimited. I express my potential more and more each day. I see problems as exciting challenges that cause me to grow stronger and stronger in faith. I vividly visualize myself as the person I want to be, and I am enthusiastically achieving my goals.

My mind is creative, and my thoughts are illuminated by the light and wisdom of God. I think the thoughts of God. Ideas are now coming to me that will help me to achieve whatever God wants in my life. I thankfully and gratefully accept these ideas and enthusiastically and immediately act on them. I radiate with power and enthusiasm. I am always positive and filled with self-confidence. I always think before I act. I control my thoughts at all times.

I have all the abilities I need to succeed. I love challenges and learn from every situation in my life. I live every day with power and passion. I feel strong, excited, passionate, and powerful. I feel tremendous confidence that I can do anything. All of my relationships are based on integrity and respect.

I awaken each day feeling healthy and alive with energy. I feel more energized throughout the day. I am bursting with energy, health, and vitality. Every pressure and tension I feel is simply a signal to relax, release, and let go. I always have more than enough energy to do all I want to do. I surrender my life to Jesus Christ. I have a wonderful, fulfilling relationship with Jesus. Jesus guides my life. I can always trust the guidance of the Holy Spirit. I feel God's presence in everything I do.

Scriptural affirmations

Therefore, having been justified by faith, we have peace with God through our Lord Jesus Christ.

—ROMANS 5:1

There is therefore now no condemnation to those who are in Christ Jesus, who do not walk according to the flesh, but according to the Spirit.

—ROMANS 8:1

Now we have received, not the spirit of the world, but the Spirit who is from God, that we might know the things that have been freely given to us by God.

—1 CORINTHIANS 2:12

For "who has known the mind of the LORD that he may instruct Him?" But we have the mind of Christ.

—1 CORINTHIANS 2:16

Or do you not know that your body is the temple of the Holy Spirit who is in you, whom you have from God, and you are not your own? For you were bought at a price; therefore glorify God in your body and in your spirit, which are God's.

—1 CORINTHIANS 6:19–20

Now He who establishes us with you in Christ and has anointed us is God.

—2 CORINTHIANS 1:21

For the love of Christ compels us, because we judge thus: that if One died for all, then all died; and He died for all, that those who live should live no longer for themselves, but for Him who died for them and rose again.

—2 CORINTHIANS 5:14–15

For He made Him who knew no sin to be sin for us, that we might become the righteousness of God in Him.

—2 CORINTHIANS 5:21

I have been crucified with Christ; it is no longer I who live, but Christ lives in me; and the life which I now live in the flesh I live by faith in the Son of God, who loved me and gave Himself for me.

—GALATIANS 2:20

Blessed be the God and Father of our Lord Jesus Christ, who has blessed us with every spiritual blessing in the heavenly places in Christ.

—EPHESIANS 1:3

That the God of our Lord Jesus Christ, the Father of glory, may give to you the spirit of wisdom and revelation in the knowledge of Him.

—EPHESIANS 1:17

Even when we were dead in trespasses, made us alive together with Christ (by grace you have been saved), and raised us up together, and made us sit together in the heavenly places in Christ Jesus.

—EPHESIANS 2:5–6

For through Him we both have access by one Spirit to the Father.

—EPHESIANS 2:18

He has delivered us from the power of darkness and conveyed us into the kingdom of the Son of His love, in whom we have redemption through His blood, the forgiveness of sins.

—COLOSSIANS 1:13–14

To them God willed to make known what are the riches of the glory of this mystery among the Gentiles: which is Christ in you, the hope of glory.

—COLOSSIANS 1:27

And you are complete in Him, who is the head of all principality and power.

—COLOSSIANS 2:10

Buried with Him in baptism, in which you also were raised with Him through faith in the working of God, who raised Him from the dead. And you, being dead in your trespasses and the uncircumcision of your flesh, He has made alive together with Him, having forgiven you all trespasses.

—COLOSSIANS 2:12–13

If then you were raised with Christ, seek those things which are above, where Christ is, sitting at the right hand of God. Set your mind on things above, not on things on the earth. For you died, and your life is hidden with Christ in God. When Christ who is our life appears, then you also will appear with Him in glory.

—COLOSSIANS 3:1–4

Let us therefore come boldly to the throne of grace, that we may obtain mercy and find grace to help in time of need.

—HEBREWS 4:16

By which have been given to us exceedingly great and precious promises, that through these you may be partakers of the divine nature, having escaped the corruption that is in the world through lust.

—2 PETER 1:4

Prayers to hold you fast

Dear Lord, I give You all my sleepless nights and exhausted days. You said to come to You for rest, and I ask You to help me to find rest in You. Help me to overcome fatigue and become energized to serve and worship You with my whole heart, mind, body, and strength. Empower and strengthen me to find renewal in You for my body, mind, and spirit. In Jesus's name, amen.

Dear Lord, I thank You that You have provided for my sleep. If my way of living is breaking any of Your principles of health and sound wisdom, I ask You to reveal it to me. Let my life line up in every way with Your perfect will so that I can enjoy the full benefits of Your blessed sleep. Amen.

Thank You, God, for leading me into a path of knowledge, because the footsteps of the righteous are ordered by the Lord. I confess that my sleep is sweet, and I awaken refreshed and renewed. In Jesus's name, amen.

Dear Lord, thank You that You are with me in everything that I do. Thank You for Your care and concern in my life. Help me to make all the changes I need to make to my routine in order to live in greater rest. And most of all, if ever I feel all alone in the middle of the night, allow me to feel Your presence to remind me that You're always there. Amen.

I thank You, God, that You promised me blessed, quiet, refreshing, and rejuvenating rest because You love me. Show me what lifestyle changes I need to make to walk in the blessings of Your gift of rest. Help me to develop a regular exercise routine, and help me to stick to it once I've begun. I thank You with all my heart for Your great and mighty love for me. Help me to order my life in a way that always pleases You. Amen.

Father God, I thank You for Your infinite wisdom that will help me navigate the best plan to reshape my thoughts and my sleep habits so that I can have complete and rejuvenating rest in You—mind, body, and spirit. I thank You for revealing these strategies to me. Now I pray that You will give me the strength I need to apply the right ones to my life. Give me the motivation I need to make rest a priority. In Jesus's name I pray, amen.

Dear Lord, I pray for supernatural rest that refreshes my body, mind, soul, and spirit. I choose to take Your yoke. Teach me to know You and to walk in Your wonderful ways. If ever I find myself struggling to enter Your place of rest, I pray beforehand that You meet me at the point of that struggle and give me inner peace and comfort, just as Jesus had during the storm, and that I'll make it safely to the other side. Amen.

Heavenly Father, I realize that fear does not come from You. I ask You to break the strongholds of fear, worry, and anxiety in my life. I receive the power, love, and sound mind you have promised to me in Your Word. I put my trust in You and rest in Your perfect peace, a peace that passes all human understanding. Amen.

Almighty God, You are the source of all power and strength. You have said that You give Your people strength. So I ask You to break the spirit of heaviness and weariness in my body and give me the knowledge and wisdom to eat correctly and to live well. Help me overcome fatigue and pain and become energized to serve and worship You with my whole heart, mind, body, and strength. Empower me to accomplish Your purpose and plans for my life. In You I will find my rest and strength. Amen.

Heavenly Father, help me reduce the stress in my life that robs my vitality and saps my strength. Show me how to work with more wisdom instead of working in ways that foolishly waste my strength. Fill me with Your peace and rest so that I may be renewed by Your presence and power. Thank You for giving me the peace that passes all understanding. Amen.

Heavenly Father, I know that You alone can strengthen and guide me out of fatigue and into Your strength and renewing power. I ask You for the wisdom to make right choices about reducing my stress, getting good nutrition, getting adequate sleep, and taking the right vitamins and supplements for my body. Thank You for the temple of my body that I can care for and use for Your glory and service. Fill me now with strength. Give me peace and rest that I may be renewed daily to live abundantly in Your good plans for my life. Amen.

Dear heavenly Father, You created me, and You are well aware of the pressures and emotional turmoil that surround me every day. Give me a special grace to rise up to a bold new level of faith and courage in You. God, I thank You that before my circumstances were ever set in motion, You had created a plan for my victory over them. Thank You for Your wonderful Word, which promises special protection and deliverance when I am tempted to feel overwhelmed by stressful circumstances. Thank You for making it possible for me to walk in Your divine health for my total being—body, mind, and spirit—free from the physical and emotional ravages of stress. In Jesus's name, amen.

Dear Lord, give me the discipline and motivation I need to invest faithfully in a regular program of exercise to help me manage stress and find the rest You promise me. Thank You for Your promise to strengthen me—body, mind, and spirit. Amen.

Dear Lord, I give You all of my stress-producing ways of thinking and living. Renew my mind by helping me to develop and learn new lifestyle strategies so that I may enjoy greater productivity, happiness, and peace. In Jesus's name, amen.

Building Blocks to a Better Night's Sleep

- All the effort in the world geared toward building a better life is for naught if that effort isn't first connected to the vine. Start with God—His Word, His promises, His intention for you.

- Staying connected to the vine includes mindfulness, joy, forgiveness, laughter, gratitude, confession, prayer, Scripture, and love.

Chapter 9

DR. COLBERT'S TWENTY-ONE NIGHTS OF SLEEP CHALLENGE

A RESTED LIFE IS within reach. It can be attained. Do you believe this? In this chapter I'm issuing you a challenge to discover the truth of it. It's time to put all the principles we've covered in this book into practice and see what a difference twenty-one perfect nights of sleep can make.

This challenge will combine daily intentions in the realm of nutrition, exercise, sleep, and stress management recommendations that have the potential to change your life. It incorporates Dr. Colbert–approved principles that form a balanced routine. Consider it twenty-one days to form a habit. We'll incorporate food and exercise recommendations, plus morning and evening routines to enhance alertness during the day and restfulness at night. It includes keeping a sleep journal, practicing a daily gratitude and appreciation exercise, receiving peaceful affirmations to guide you into sleep each night, and daily prayers and scriptures to keep you grounded in God.

A few recommendations before you get started:

Meet with your doctor to talk over the supplement

179

recommendations I gave in chapter 6. Let him help you discover which ones would work best for your sleep challenge.

Plan to consume three well-balanced meals—breakfast, lunch, and dinner—every day with two snacks, one midmorning and one late afternoon.

Make twenty-one copies of each of the journal and gratitude pages (found at the end of this chapter) before you begin the challenge, and keep them accessible throughout the twenty-one days.

Are you up for it? Let's get started.

DAY 1

Morning

- Eat a well-balanced breakfast.

- Complete your sleep journal entry for last night's night of sleep. (See end of chapter.)

- Exercise for thirty minutes.

Midmorning

- Enjoy one of the recommended morning snacks from chapter 6 about two to three hours after breakfast.

Midday

- Eat a well-balanced lunch.

- Fill out your gratitude/appreciation journal for the day. (See end of chapter.)

Midafternoon

- Enjoy one of the recommended evening snacks from chapter 6 about two to three hours after lunch.

Evening

- Eat a well-balanced dinner.

- Take the sleep-conducive supplement or natural sleep aid approved by your doctor.

- Drink a cup of Sleepytime Tea.

- Remove electronics from the bedroom and close the shades.

- Pray an evening Scripture affirmation: "IIn peace I will lie down and sleep, for you alone, O Lord, will keep me safe" (Ps. 4:8).

- Go to bed at a predetermined time to ensure seven to nine hours of sleep.

DAY 2

Morning

- Eat a well-balanced breakfast.

- Complete your sleep journal entry for last night's night of sleep.

- Create a simple to-do list that lists the three most important priorities for the day.

Midmorning

- Enjoy one of the recommended morning snacks from chapter 6 about two to three hours after breakfast.

Midday

- Eat a well-balanced lunch.

- Fill out your gratitude/appreciation journal for the day.

- Eat four rice cakes for a midday snack.

Midafternoon

- Enjoy one of the recommended evening snacks from chapter 6 about two to three hours after lunch.

Evening

- Eat a well-balanced dinner.

- Take a bath with Epsom salts.

- Tidy up the bedroom, removing storage boxes and putting away piles of clothes.

- Pray an evening Scripture affirmation: "It is vain for you to rise up early, to sit up late, to eat the bread of sorrows; for so He gives His beloved sleep" (Ps. 127:2).

- Go to bed at a predetermined time to ensure seven to nine hours of sleep.

Day 3

Morning

- Eat a well-balanced breakfast.

- Complete your sleep journal entry for last night's night of sleep.

- Exercise for thirty minutes.

Midmorning

- Enjoy one of the recommended morning snacks from chapter 6 about two to three hours after breakfast.

Midday

- Eat a well-balanced lunch.

- Fill out your gratitude/appreciation journal for the day.

Midafternoon

- Enjoy one of the recommended evening snacks from chapter 6 about two to three hours after lunch.

Evening

- Eat a well-balanced dinner.

- Take the sleep-conducive supplement or natural sleep aid approved by your doctor.

- Stop using screens (TV, computer, phone) an hour before bed.

- Pray an evening Scripture affirmation: "You can go to bed without fear; you will lie down and sleep soundly" (Prov. 3:24, NLT).

- Go to bed at a predetermined time to ensure seven to nine hours of sleep.

Day 4

Morning

- Eat a well-balanced breakfast.

- Complete your sleep journal entry for last night's night of sleep.

- Review the list of ten distortional thoughts (refer to chapter 7) and determine which one is plaguing you most right now. Consider how you might reframe it in light of a current circumstance.

Midmorning

- Enjoy one of the recommended morning snacks from chapter 6 about two to three hours after breakfast.

Midday

- Eat a well-balanced lunch.

- Fill out your gratitude/appreciation journal for the day.

Midafternoon

- Enjoy one of the recommended evening snacks from chapter 6 about two to three hours after lunch.

Evening

- Eat a well-balanced dinner.

- Take the sleep-conducive supplement or natural sleep aid approved by your doctor.

- Evaluate the quality of your pillow and mattress to determine if they need to be replaced.

- Pray an evening Scripture affirmation: "You will keep him in perfect peace, whose mind is stayed on You, because he trusts in You" (Isa. 26:3).

- Go to bed at a predetermined time to ensure seven to nine hours of sleep.

Day 5

Morning

- Eat a well-balanced breakfast.

- Complete your sleep journal entry for last night's night of sleep.

- Exercise for thirty minutes.

Midmorning

- Enjoy one of the recommended morning snacks from chapter 6 about two to three hours after breakfast.

Midday

- Eat a well-balanced lunch.

- Fill out your gratitude/appreciation journal for the day.

- Treat yourself to a nap.

Midafternoon

- Enjoy one of the recommended evening snacks from chapter 6 about two to three hours after lunch.

Evening

- Eat a well-balanced dinner.

- Take the sleep-conducive supplement or natural sleep aid approved by your doctor.

- Choose not to watch or read the evening news.

- Pray an evening Scripture affirmation: "Then Jesus said, 'Come to me, all of you who are weary and carry heavy burdens, and I will give you rest'" (Matt. 11:28, NLT).

- Go to bed at a predetermined time to ensure seven to nine hours of sleep.

DAY 6

Morning

- Eat a well-balanced breakfast.

- Complete your sleep journal entry for last night's night of sleep.

- Review a big project that's on your plate right now. What are the major steps you need to take to complete it? Write them down, then label them in the order they need to be completed. Pick one step you can take toward the first piece of the project today and be sure to complete it.

Midmorning

- Enjoy one of the recommended morning snacks from chapter 6 about two to three hours after breakfast.

Midday

- Eat a well-balanced lunch.

- Fill out your gratitude/appreciation journal for the day.

Midafternoon

- Enjoy one of the recommended evening snacks from chapter 6 about two to three hours after lunch.

Evening

- Eat a well-balanced dinner.

- Take the sleep-conducive supplement or natural sleep aid approved by your doctor.

- Evaluate your bedroom. What else needs to be done to make it a safe haven for sleep? What step can you take to make it so?

- Pray an evening Scripture affirmation: "[Jesus said,] 'Peace I leave with you, My peace I give to you; not as the world gives do I give to you. Let not your heart be troubled, neither let it be afraid'" (John 14:27).

- Go to bed at a predetermined time to ensure seven to nine hours of sleep.

Day 7

Morning

- Eat a well-balanced breakfast.

- Complete your sleep journal entry for last night's night of sleep.

- Exercise for thirty minutes.

Midmorning

- Enjoy one of the recommended morning snacks from chapter 6 about two to three hours after breakfast.

Midday

- Eat a well-balanced lunch.

- Fill out your gratitude/appreciation journal for the day.

Midafternoon

- Enjoy one of the recommended evening snacks from chapter 6 about two to three hours after lunch.

Evening

- Eat a well-balanced dinner.

- Take the sleep-conducive supplement or natural sleep aid approved by your doctor.

- Pray an evening Scripture affirmation: "Casting down arguments and every high thing that exalts itself against the knowledge of God, bringing every thought into captivity to the obedience of Christ" (2 Cor. 10:5).

- Go to bed at a predetermined time to ensure seven to nine hours of sleep.

DAY 8

Morning

- Complete your sleep journal entry for last night's night of sleep.

- Review your daily caffeine intake. In light of the information shared in chapter 3 regarding caffeine, what adjustments, if any, do you need to make to your caffeine consumption? Will you commit to this?

Midmorning

- Enjoy one of the recommended morning snacks from chapter 6 about two to three hours after breakfast.

Midday

- Eat a well-balanced lunch.

- Fill out your gratitude/appreciation journal for the day.

- Take time to think about the "six months to live" test (see chapter 8). If you had six months left to live, what would be most important to you?

Midafternoon

- Enjoy one of the recommended evening snacks from chapter 6 about two to three hours after lunch.

Evening

- Eat a well-balanced dinner.

- Take sleep-conducive supplement.

- Enjoy a cup of Sleepytime Tea before bed.

- Pray an evening Scripture affirmation: "Be anxious for nothing, but in everything by prayer and supplication, with thanksgiving, let your requests be made known to God; and the peace of God, which surpasses all understanding, will guard your hearts and minds through Christ Jesus" (Phil. 4:6–7).

- Go to bed at a predetermined time to ensure seven to nine hours of sleep.

DAY 9

Morning

- Eat a well-balanced breakfast.

- Complete your sleep journal entry for last night's night of sleep.

- Exercise for thirty minutes.

Midmorning

- Enjoy one of the recommended morning snacks from chapter 6 about two to three hours after breakfast.

Midday

- Eat a well-balanced lunch.

- Fill out your gratitude/appreciation journal for the day.

Midafternoon

- Enjoy one of the recommended evening snacks from chapter 6 about two to three hours after lunch.

Evening

- Eat a well-balanced dinner.

- Take the sleep-conducive supplement or natural sleep aid approved by your doctor.

- Do noises inside or outside your home environment keep you from restful sleep? Consider whether to purchase a pair of earplugs.

- Pray an evening Scripture affirmation: "For God has not given [me] a spirit of fear, but of power and of love and of a sound mind" (2 Tim. 1:7).

- Go to bed at a predetermined time to ensure seven to nine hours of sleep.

DAY 10

Morning

- Eat a well-balanced breakfast.

- Complete your sleep journal entry for last night's night of sleep.

- Review whether there any physical conditions—an injury, snoring habits, weight gain, night terrors, or sleepwalking, perhaps—that could be contributing to poor sleep for you. Does the condition require a doctor's review? If so, make an appointment today.

Midmorning

- Enjoy one of the recommended morning snacks from chapter 6 about two to three hours after breakfast.

Midday

- Eat a well-balanced lunch.

- Fill out your gratitude/appreciation journal for the day.

- Purchase earplugs, if necessary.

Midafternoon

- Enjoy one of the recommended evening snacks from chapter 6 about two to three hours after lunch.

Evening

- Eat a well-balanced dinner.

- Take sleep-conducive supplement.

- Consider the sources of sugar in your diet. Do you need to reduce your intake of sugar? How can you commit to doing so? What foods will you put in its place?

- Pray an evening Scripture affirmation: "For only we who believe can enter his rest" (Heb. 4:3, NLT).

- Go to bed at a predetermined time to ensure seven to nine hours of sleep.

Day 11

Morning

- Eat a well-balanced breakfast.

- Complete your sleep journal entry for last night's night of sleep.

- Exercise for thirty minutes.

Midmorning

- Enjoy one of the recommended morning snacks from chapter 6 about two to three hours after breakfast.

Midday

- Eat a well-balanced lunch.

- Fill out your gratitude/appreciation journal for the day.

- Spend your lunch hour outside under a shade tree.

Midafternoon

- Enjoy one of the recommended evening snacks from chapter 6 about two to three hours after lunch.

Evening

- Eat a well-balanced dinner.

- Take sleep-conducive supplement.

- Take a bath with lavender oil.

- Pray an evening Scripture affirmation: "The sleep of the working man is pleasant, whether he eats little or much; but the full stomach of the rich man does not allow him to sleep" (Eccles. 5:12, NAS).

- Go to bed at a predetermined time to ensure seven to nine hours of sleep.

DAY 12

Morning

- Eat a well-balanced breakfast.

- Complete your sleep journal entry for last night's night of sleep.

- Take a moment to reflect on the progress of this twenty-one-day challenge so far. What have been the benefits? What has been challenging?

Midmorning

- Enjoy one of the recommended morning snacks from chapter 6 about two to three hours after breakfast.

Midday

- Eat a well-balanced lunch.

- Fill out your gratitude/appreciation journal for the day.

- Review your usual alcohol intake in light of the perspective offered in chapter 3. Do you need to adjust your consumption? What commitment will you make regarding this?

Midafternoon

- Enjoy one of the recommended evening snacks from chapter 6 about two to three hours after lunch.

Evening

- Eat a well-balanced dinner.

- Take sleep-conducive supplement.

- Enjoy a serving of low-fat whole-grain crackers with a teaspoon of peanut butter before bed.

- Pray an evening Scripture affirmation: "Casting all your care upon Him, for He cares for you" (1 Pet. 5:7).

- Go to bed at a predetermined time to ensure seven to nine hours of sleep.

Day 13

Morning

- Eat a well-balanced breakfast.

- Complete your sleep journal entry for last night's night of sleep.

- Exercise for thirty minutes.

Midmorning

- Enjoy one of the recommended morning snacks from chapter 6 about two to three hours after breakfast.

Midday

- Eat a well-balanced lunch.

- Fill out your gratitude/appreciation journal for the day.

- Spend your lunch hour being fully attentive to the present moment, practicing mindfulness (see chapter 8).

Evening

- Eat a well-balanced dinner.

- Take sleep-conducive supplement.

- Dim the lights in your home as the sun begins to go down in the sky.

- Pray an evening Scripture affirmation: "For I have given rest to the weary and joy to the sorrowing" (Jer. 31:25, NLT).

- Go to bed at a predetermined time to ensure seven to nine hours of sleep.

Day 14

Morning

- Eat a well-balanced breakfast.

- Complete your sleep journal entry for last night's night of sleep.

- Take a few moments to think about the presence of faith in your life right now. In what ways is your faith being exercised? How might God be inviting more faith from you?

Midmorning

- Enjoy one of the recommended morning snacks from chapter 6 about two to three hours after breakfast.

Midday

- Eat a well-balanced lunch.

- Fill out your gratitude/appreciation journal for the day.

- Treat yourself to a massage.

Midafternoon

- Enjoy one of the recommended evening snacks from chapter 6 about two to three hours after lunch.

Evening

- Eat a well-balanced dinner.

- Take sleep-conducive supplement.

- Use your bed only for sleep activities tonight—no reading, snacking, working, or worrying in bed.

- Pray an evening Scripture affirmation: "For 'who has known the mind of the Lord that he may instruct Him?' But we have the mind of Christ" (1 Cor. 2:16).

- Go to bed at a predetermined time to ensure seven to nine hours of sleep.

DAY 15

Morning

- Eat a well-balanced breakfast.

- Complete your sleep journal entry for last night's night of sleep.

- Exercise for thirty minutes.

Midmorning

- Enjoy one of the recommended morning snacks from chapter 6 about two to three hours after breakfast.

Midday

- Eat a well-balanced lunch.

- Fill out your gratitude/appreciation journal for the day.

- Take a nap today.

Midafternoon

- Enjoy one of the recommended evening snacks from chapter 6 about two to three hours after lunch.

Evening

- Eat a well-balanced dinner.

- Take sleep-conducive supplement.

- Keep your portion size reasonable at dinner.

- Pray an evening Scripture affirmation: "Or do you not know that your body is the temple of the Holy Spirit who is in you, whom you have from God, and you are not your own? For you were bought at a price; therefore glorify God in your body and in your spirit, which are God's" (1 Cor. 6:19–20).

- Go to bed at a predetermined time to ensure seven to nine hours of sleep.

Day 16

Morning

- Eat a well-balanced breakfast.

- Complete your sleep journal entry for last night's night of sleep.

- What worries are on your mind today? Spend time trusting those worries into the care of God.

Midmorning

- Enjoy one of the recommended morning snacks from chapter 6 about two to three hours after breakfast.

Midday

- Eat a well-balanced lunch.

- Fill out your gratitude/appreciation journal for the day.

- Spend time reflecting on the ways love is showing up—or not showing up—in you right now. How can you practice being even more loving?

Midafternoon

- Enjoy one of the recommended evening snacks from chapter 6 about two to three hours after lunch.

Evening

- Eat a well-balanced dinner.

- Take sleep-conducive supplement.

- How is the temperature in your room? Do you need to incorporate a fan or better venting system?

- Pray an evening Scripture affirmation: "I am leaving you with a gift—peace of mind and heart" (John 14:27, NLT).

- Go to bed at a predetermined time to ensure seven to nine hours of sleep.

DAY 17

Morning

- Eat a well-balanced breakfast.

- Complete your sleep journal entry for last night's night of sleep.

- Exercise for thirty minutes.

Midmorning

- Enjoy one of the recommended morning snacks from chapter 6 about two to three hours after breakfast.

Midday

- Eat a well-balanced lunch.

- Fill out your gratitude/appreciation journal for the day.

- Think about your next day off, and give yourself permission to treat it like a Sabbath. Make a list of the kinds of relaxing activities you will do on that day.

Midafternoon

- Enjoy one of the recommended evening snacks from chapter 6 about two to three hours after lunch.

Evening

- Eat a well-balanced dinner.

- Take sleep-conducive supplement.

- Listen to soothing music before bed.

- Pray an evening Scripture affirmation: "Blessed be the God and Father of our Lord Jesus Christ, who has blessed us with every spiritual blessing in the heavenly places in Christ" (Eph. 1:3).

- Go to bed at a predetermined time to ensure seven to nine hours of sleep.

Day 18

Morning

- Eat a well-balanced breakfast.

- Complete your sleep journal entry for last night's night of sleep.

- Consider what is creating the greatest amount of stress in your life at the moment. What can be changed about the situation, either in terms of reframing or making a better choice?

Midmorning

- Enjoy one of the recommended morning snacks from chapter 6 about two to three hours after breakfast.

Midday

- Eat a well-balanced lunch.

- Fill out your gratitude/appreciation journal for the day.

- Do several stretching exercises.

Midafternoon

- Enjoy one of the recommended evening snacks from chapter 6 about two to three hours after lunch.

Evening

- Eat a well-balanced dinner.

- Take sleep-conducive supplement.

- Practice abdominal breathing.

- Pray an evening Scripture affirmation: "If then you were raised with Christ, seek those things which are above, where Christ is, sitting at the right hand of God. Set your mind on things above, not on things on the earth. For you died, and your life is hidden with Christ in God. When Christ who is our life appears, then you also will appear with Him in glory" (Col. 3:1–4).

- Go to bed at a predetermined time to ensure seven to nine hours of sleep.

DAY 19

Morning

- Eat a well-balanced breakfast.

- Complete your sleep journal entry for last night's night of sleep.

- Exercise for thirty minutes.

Midmorning

- Enjoy one of the recommended morning snacks from chapter 6 about two to three hours after breakfast.

Midday

- Eat a well-balanced lunch.

- Fill out your gratitude/appreciation journal for the day.

Midafternoon

- Enjoy one of the recommended evening snacks from chapter 6 about two to three hours after lunch.

Evening

- Eat a well-balanced dinner.

- Take sleep-conducive supplement.

- Share funny stories with a loved one to get yourself laughing.

- Pray an evening Scripture affirmation: "Let us therefore come boldly to the throne of grace, that we may obtain mercy and find grace to help in time of need" (Heb. 4:16).

- Go to bed at a predetermined time to ensure seven to nine hours of sleep.

Day 20

Morning

- Eat a well-balanced breakfast.

- Complete your sleep journal entry for last night's night of sleep.

- Review the ten distortional thoughts (see chapter 7). Which one is at work in your mind on this particular day? How can you reframe it into a healthier mind-set?

Midmorning

- Enjoy one of the recommended morning snacks from chapter 6 about two to three hours after breakfast.

Midday

- Eat a well-balanced lunch.

- Fill out your gratitude/appreciation journal for the day.

Midafternoon

- Enjoy one of the recommended evening snacks from chapter 6 about two to three hours after lunch.

Evening

- Eat a well-balanced dinner.

- Practice progressive muscle relaxation before bed.

- Pray an evening Scripture affirmation: "There remaineth therefore a rest to the people of God" (Heb. 4:9, KJV).

- Go to bed at a predetermined time to ensure seven to nine hours of sleep.

Day 21

Morning

- Eat a well-balanced breakfast.

- Complete your sleep journal entry for last night's night of sleep.

- Exercise for thirty minutes.

Midmorning

- Enjoy one of the recommended morning snacks from chapter 6 about two to three hours after breakfast.

Midday

- Eat a well-balanced lunch.

- Fill out your gratitude/appreciation journal for the day.

- Treat yourself a nap today.

Midafternoon

- Enjoy one of the recommended evening snacks from chapter 6 about two to three hours after lunch.

Evening

- Eat a well-balanced dinner.

- Take sleep-conducive supplement.

- Spend time in a visualization exercise before bed, imagining yourself in the most calming environment you can imagine.

- Pray an evening Scripture affirmation: "Indeed, he who watches over Israel never slumbers or sleeps" (Ps. 121:4, NLT). Go to bed at a predetermined time to ensure seven to nine hours of sleep.

SLEEP JOURNAL

Day	Bedtime	Wake-Up Time	No. of Hours Slept	I Felt . . .	Notes
1					
2					
3					
4					
5					
6					
7					
8					
9					
10					
11					
12					
13					
14					
15					
16					
17					

Day	Bedtime	Wake-Up Time	No. of Hours Slept	I Felt . . .	Notes
18					
19					
20					
21					

GRATITUDE/APPRECIATION JOURNAL

Day	Today I Am Thankful for...
1	
2	
3	
4	
5	
6	
7	
8	
9	
10	
11	
12	
13	
14	
15	
16	
17	
18	

Day	Today I Am Thankful for...
19	
20	
21	

The Verdict Is In

So, how was this three-week challenge for you? Did you incorporate behaviors that have become new habits? Has your sleep improved? Do you feel more rested? Have you found a rhythm of life that fosters greater rest and ease?

Remember that the goal is to turn our lives over to God in a way that leaves us "rest assured" on a daily basis. It takes a combination of slowing, mindfulness, healthy eating, exercise, and intention to bring this about. It is the life God has for you! Keep claiming it each and every day—leading to calm and restful nights. Rest assured!

RESOURCES FOR SLEEP DISORDERS

Divine Health nutritional products
   1908 Boothe Circle
   Longwood, FL 32750
   Phone: (407) 331-7007
   Web Site: www.drcolbert.com
   E-mail: info@drcolbert.com

Comprehensive multivitamin
   Divine Health Living Multivitamin and Divine Health Multivitamin

Sleep support

- Amino acids: Divine Health 5-HTP, Divine Health Serotonin Max, L-Theanine, GABA, TryptoPure

- Melatonin: Divine Health Melatonin (1 mg and 3 mg)

- Magnesium: Natural Calm, Divine Health Chelated Magnesium

- Adaptogens: Divine Health Stress Manager (magnolia bark), Divine Health Relora Plus

- Sleep herbs: Divine Health Sleep Formula

From health food store
   Chamomile tea and Sleepytime Tea

NOTES

INTRODUCTION
THE RED BULL GENERATION

1. Tim Chen, "American Household Credit Card Debt Statistics: 2014," http://www.nerdwallet.com/blog/credit-card-data/average-credit-card-debt-household/ (accessed March 11, 2015).

2. Ibid.

3. Dave Ramsey, *The Total Money Makeover* (Nashville, TN: Thomas Nelson Inc., 2003), 23.

4. Paul Pearsall, *Toxic Success* (Makawao, HI: Inner Ocean Publishing, 2002), 68; see also Divorce Rates, http://www.divorcereform.org/rates.html (accessed January 2, 2015).

5. David Hinckley, "Average American Watches 5 Hours of TV Per Day, Report Shows, " *Daily News*, http://www.nydailynews.com/life-style/average-american-watches-5-hours-tv-day-article-1.1711954 (accessed January 2, 2009).

6. Doc Childre and Deborah Rozman, *Overcoming Emotional Chaos* (San Diego, CA: Jodere Group Inc., 2002), 226.

7. Division of Sleep Medicine at Harvard Medical School, "Judgment and Safety," http://healthysleep.med.harvard .edu/need-sleep/whats-in-it-for-you/judgment-safety#2 (accessed January 2, 2015).

CHAPTER 1
WHY DO I NEED TO SLEEP?

1. CNN.com, "Lack of Sleep America's Top Health Problem, Doctors Say," Health Story Page, March 17, 1997, http://www.cnn.com/HEALTH/9703/17/nfm/sleep .deprivation/ (accessed January 2, 2015).

2. CNN.com Transcripts, "Clinton Pardons: House Government Reform Committee Questions Former Clinton Aides," Special Event, aired March 1, 2001, http:// transcripts.cnn.com/TRANSCRIPTS/0103/01/se.16 .html (accessed January 2, 2015).

3. Jeanne Wright, "A Short Trip From Fatigue to Felony," *Los Angeles Times*, February 16, 2005, http://articles. latimes.com/2005/feb/16/autos/hy-wheels16 (accessed January 2, 2015).

4. Lawrence J. Epstein and Steven Mardon, *The Harvard Medical School Guide to a Good Night's Sleep* (New York: McGraw-Hill, 2007), 4.

5. Ibid., 5.

6. Ibid., 4.

7. Insomnia911.com, "Insomnia Statistics," http://www .insomnia911.com/insomnia-facts/statistics.htm (accessed January 2, 2015).

8. National Heart Lung and Blood Institute, "Insomnia: Who Is at Risk for Insomnia?", Insomnia in Women and African Americans, http://www.nhlbi.nih.gov/ health/health-topics/topics/inso/atrisk (accessed January 2, 2015).

9. Insomnia911.com, "Insomnia Statistics."

10. Ibid.

11. Ibid.

12. Ibid.

13. Delta Sleep Labs, "Facts and Statistics," http:// deltasleeplabs.com/Facts_and_Statistics.html (accessed January 2, 2015)

14. Ibid.

15. Ibid.

16. Gregg D. Jacobs, *Say Good Night to Insomnia* (New York: Henry Holt and Company, LLC, 1998), 21.

17. Texas Sleep Medicine, "Insomnia," http://www .txsleepmedicine.com/department/insomnia/ (accessed January 5, 2015).

18. Committee on Sleep Medicine and Research, *Sleep Disorders and Sleep Deprivation: An Unmet Public Health Problem*, The Institute of Medicine, April 4, 2006, press release, http://www.iom.edu/reports/2006/ sleep-disorders-and-sleep-deprivation-an-unmet -public-health-problem.aspx (accessed January 5, 2015).

19. Stephanie Saul, "Record Sales of Sleeping Pills Are Causing Worries," *New York Times*, February 7, 2006, http://www.nytimes.com/2006/02/07/business/07sleep

.html?ex=1156305600&en=b3db11459ac65eff&ei=5070 (accessed January 5, 2015).

20. National Sleep Foundation, "2000 Omnibus Sleep in America Poll,"1522 K Street NW, Suite 500, Washington, DC, 20005.

21. Ibid.

22. Kelly Myers, lecture notes for Psyc 2000 001, Louisiana State University, August 30, 2001, http://chancely29 .tripod.com/lsunotes/id2.html (accessed January 5, 2015).

23. American Psychological Association, "Why Sleep Is Important and What Happens When You Don't Get Enough," http://www.apa.org/topics/whysleep.html (accessed January 5, 2015).

24. Ibid.

25. K. Spiegle, R. Leproult, and E. Van Cauter, "Impact of Sleep Debt on Metabolic and Endocrine Function," *Lancet* 354 (October 23, 1999): 1435–1439, referenced in "Backgrounder: Why Sleep Matters," http://sleep foundation.org/how-sleep-works/how-much-sleep-do -we-really-need/page/0%2C1/ (accessed January 5, 2015).

26. Epstein, *The Harvard Medical School Guide to a Good Night's Sleep*, 6.

27. Ibid., 35.

28. A. A. Kuo, "Does Sleep Deprivation Impair Cognitive and Motor Performance as Much as Alcohol Intoxication?" *Western Journal of Medicine* 3, no. 174 (March 1, 2001): 180, referenced in "Backgrounder: Why Sleep

Matters," http://www.sleepfoundation.org/NSAW/pk_
background.cfm (accessed February 10, 2005).

29. Stephenie Overman, "Rise and Sigh—Sleep Deprivation," *HR Magazine*, May 1999, http://www.findarticles
.com/p/articles/mi_m3495/is_5_44/ai_54711192
(accessed February 16, 2006).

30. Summary of Findings, National Sleep Foundation 2005
Sleep in America Poll.

31. *APA Online*, "Why Sleep Is Important and What Happens When You Don't Get Enough," http://www.apa
.org/topics/sleep/why.aspx (accessed January 5, 2015).

32. Shawn M. Talbott, PhD, *The Cortisol Connection*
(Alameda, CA: Hunter House 2002), 52–54.

33. Don Colbert, "7 Pillars of Health" PowerPoint pre-
sentation; also, Summary of Findings, National Sleep
Foundation 2005 Sleep in America Poll.

34. Circadian Technologies, Inc., "5 Negative Effects of
High Overtime Levels," 2014 Health Study Release,
http://www.circadian.com/blog/item/22-5-negative
-effects-of-high-overtime-levels.html?tmpl=component
&print=1#.VKrE3yvF-So (accessed January 5, 2015).

35. WebMD.com, "Physical Side Effects of Oversleeping,"
Sleep Disorders Health Center, http://www.webmd.com/
sleep-disorders/guide/physical-side-effects-oversleeping
(accessed January 5, 2015).

36. Ibid.

37. Ibid.

38. WebMD.com, "Older Women's Stroke Risk Linked to Sleep," Stroke Health Center, http://www.webmd.com/stroke/news/20080717/older-womens-stroke-risk-linked-to-sleep (accessed January 5, 2015).

39. Maria Thomas et al., "Neural Basis of Alertness and Cognitive Performance Impairments During Sleepiness: I. Effects of 24 h of Sleep Deprivation on Waking Human Regional Brain Activity," *Journal of Sleep Research* 9, no. 4 (December 2000): 335–352.

40. Summary of Findings, National Sleep Foundation 2005 Sleep in America Poll, http://sleepfoundation.org/sites/default/files/2005_summary_of_findings.pdf (accessed January 5, 2015).

CHAPTER 2
THE ARCHITECTURE OF SLEEP

1. National Sleep Foundation, http://sleepfoundation.org/how-sleep-works/how-much-sleep-do-we-really-need (accessed January 5, 2015).

2. Anna H. Wu, Renwei Wang, Woon-Puay Koh, et al., "Sleep Duration, Melatonin, and Breast Cancer Among Chinese Women in Singapore," *Carcinogenesis* 29, no. 6 (2008): 1244–1248, http://carcin.oxfordjournals.org/cgi/content/full/29/6/1244 (accessed January 5, 2015).

3. Ron Chepesiuk, "Missing the Dark: Health Effects of Light Pollution," *Environmental Health Perspectives* 117, no. 1 (January 2009), http://ehp.niehs.nih.gov/117-a20/ (accessed January 5, 2015).

4. Press Release, "IARC Monographs Programme Finds Cancer Hazards Associated With Shiftwork, Painting and Firefighting," The International Agency for Research on Cancer, December 5, 2007, http://www .iarc.fr/en/media-centre/pr/2007/pr180.html (accessed January 5, 2015).

5. Russel Reiter, University of Texas, "Increase in childhood leukaemia may be due to increased light at night," Children With Leukemia, September 2004, http://www.childrenwithcancer.org.uk/News/increase-in-childhood-leukaemia-may-be-due-to-increased-light-at-night (accessed August 12, 2009).

CHAPTER 3
WHAT'S ROBBING YOU OF A GOOD NIGHT'S SLEEP?

1. Gregg D. Jacobs, "Lifestyle Practices That Can Improve Sleep (Part 2)," Talk About Sleep, http://www.talk aboutsleep.com/lifestyle-practices-that-can-improve -sleep-part-ii (accessed January 6, 2015).

2. Max Hirshkowitz and Patricia B. Smith, *Sleep Disorders for Dummies* (Hoboken, NJ: Wiley Publishing Inc., 2004), 184.

3. The Sleep Well, "Radio Frequency (RF) Procedure or Somnoplasty," Sleep Apnea Information and Resources, http://www.stanford.edu/~dement/apnea.html (accessed January 6, 2015).

4. Don Colbert, "7 Pillars of Health."

5. Some points in this list have been adapted from University of Maryland Medical Center, "Insomnia—Treatment: Sleep Hygiene Tips."

Chapter 4
Sleep Disorders

1. American Psychological Association, "Why Sleep Is Important and What Happens When You Don't Get Enough."

2. National Heart Lung and Blood Institute "What Is Insomnia?" US Department of Health and Human Service, http://www.nhlbi.nih.gov/health/dci/Diseases/inso/inso_whatis.html (accessed August 11, 2009).

3. SleepMedInc.com, "Sleep Disorders: Sleep Statistics," http://www2.sleepmedinc.com/page/1896 (accessed March 11, 2015).

4. H. Klar Yaggi, John Concato, Walter N. Kernan, et al., "Obstructive Sleep Apnea as a Risk Factor for Stroke and Death," *New England Journal of Medicine* 353, no. 19 (November 10, 2005): 2034–2041, abstract viewed at http://content.nejm.org/cgi/content/short/353/19/2034 (accessed January 6, 2015).

5. Associated Press, "Sleep Apnea May Have Contributed to Death," ESPN.com, December 28, 2004, http://sports.espn.go.com/nfl/news/story?id=1953876 (accessed January 6, 2015).

6. Carlos H. Schenck, *Sleep* (New York: Avery, 2008), 36.

7. American Sleep Association, "Sleep Apnea," http://www.sleepassociation.org/patients-general-public/

sleep-apnea/what-is-sleep-apnea/ (accessed January 6, 2015).

8. Medline Plus, "Obstructive Sleep Apnea," http://www .nlm.nih.gov/medlineplus/ency/article/000811.htm (accessed January 6, 2015).

9. SleepMedInc.com, "Sleep Disorders: Sleep Statistics."

10. National Institute of Neurological Disorders and Stroke, "Narcolepsy Fact Sheet," http://www.ninds.nih.gov/ disorders/narcolepsy/detail_narcolepsy.htm#58833201 (accessed January 6, 2015).

11. Epstein, *The Harvard Medical School Guide to a Good Night's Sleep*, 157.

12. Ibid.

13. National Institute of Neurological Disorders and Stroke, "Restless Legs Syndrome Fact Sheet," http://www.ninds .nih.gov/disorders/restless_legs/detail_restless_legs.htm (accessed January 6, 2015).

14. Epstein, *The Harvard Medical School Guide to a Good Night's Sleep*, 147.

15. Herbert Ross with Keri Brenner, *Alternative Medicine Magazine's Definitive Guide to Sleep Disorders* (Berkeley, CA: Celestial Arts, 2000, 2007), 27.

16. Hirshkowitz and Smith, *Sleep Disorders for Dummies*, 254.

17. Epstein, *The Harvard Medical School Guide to a Good Night's Sleep*, 171.

18. Ibid., 169.

19. Hirshkowitz and Smith, *Sleep Disorders for Dummies*, 237–238.

20. Epstein, *The Harvard Medical School Guide to a Good Night's Sleep*, 179.

21. Ibid., 172–173.

22. Ibid., 173–174.

CHAPTER 5
PROACTIVE SLEEP THERAPIES

1. Hara Estroff Marano, "New Light on Seasonal Depression," *Psychology Today*, November 1, 2003, http://www.psychologytoday.com/articles/200311/new-light-seasonal-depression (accessed January 6, 2015).

2. For more information about full-spectrum lights or light boxes, call the SunBox Company at (800) 548-3968 or Environmental Lighting Concepts, Inc. (OttLite Technology) at (301) 869-5980.

3. S. Lynne Walker, "More Americans Are Waking Up to the Benefits of Midday Snooze," SignOnSanDiego.com, September 4, 2007, http://www.signonsandiego.com/news/nation/20070924-9999-1n24sleep.html (accessed January 6, 2015).

4. University of Maryland Medical Center, "Insomnia—Treatment: Behavioral Therapy Methods," http://www.umm.edu/patiented/articles/what_behavioral_other_non-drug_treatments_insomnia_000027_7.htm (accessed August 12, 2009).

5. Edmund Jacobson, *Progressive Relaxation*, 3rd rev. ed. (Chicago, IL: University of Chicago Press, 1974).

6. "Progressive Relaxation," http://www.mindspring
.com/~yepstein/progrel.htm (accessed April 13, 2005).

7. Robert Woolfolk and Frank Richardson, *Stress, Sanity, and Survival* (New York: Signet Books, 1979).

8. Rick Warren, *The Purpose Driven Life* (Grand Rapids, MI: Zondervan, 2002), 90.

9. "Techniques: Everything You Wanted to Know About Massage," AboutMassage.Com, http://aboutmassage
.com/techniques/ (accessed April 13, 2005).

10. Ibid.

Chapter 6
Healthy Lifestyle Changes for
a Better Night's Sleep

1. Barry Sears, *Omega Rx Zone* (New York: Harper Collins, 2002).

2. I. V. Zhdanova, R. J. Wurtman, H. J. Lynch, et al., "Sleep-Inducing Effects of Low Doses of Melatonin Ingested in the Evening," *Clinical Pharmacology and Therapeutics* 57, no. 5 (May 1995): 552–558, http://www
.ncbi.nlm.nih.gov/pubmed/7768078 (accessed January 7, 2015).

3. Discover Nutrition, "Rapid Anxiety and Stress Relief," http://www.discovernutrition.com/l-theanine.html (accessed January 7, 2015).

4. Aeron Lifecycles Clinical Laboratory, "Sleepless Night, Irritable Days, and Fatigue? It Could Be Your Hormones," *Hormonal Update* 2, no. 12, http://www.aeron

.com/volume_2_number_12.htm (accessed August 12, 2009).

5. O. Picazo and A. Fernández-Guasti, "Anti-Anxiety Effects of Progesterone and Some of Its Reduced Metabolites: An Evaluation Using the Burying Behavior Test," *Brain Research* 680, nos. 1–2 (1995): 135–141, http://www.biomedexperts.com/Abstract.bme/7663969/ Anti-anxiety_effects_of_progesterone_and_some_of_ its_reduced_metabolites_an_evaluation_using_the_ burying_behavior_test (accessed January 7, 2015).

6. A. H. Soderpalm, S. Lindsey, R. H. Purdy, et al., "Administration of Progesterone Produces Mild Sedative-Like Effects in Men and Women," *Psychoneuroendocrinology* 29, no. 3 (April 2004): 339–354.

7. "Hatha Yoga and Its Effects," SelfGrowth.com, http:// www.selfgrowth.com/articles/Various1.html (accessed January 7, 2015).

8. Marian S. Garfinkel, et al., "Yoga-Based Intervention for Carpal Tunnel Syndrome," *Journal of the American Medical Association* 280 (November 11, 1998): 1601– 1603.

9. P. Jin, "Changes in Heart Rate, Noradrenaline, Cortisol and Mood During Tai Chi," *Journal of Psychosomatic Research* 33 (1989): 197–206.

CHAPTER 7
PUTTING STRESS, ANXIETY, FEAR, AND WORRY TO BED

1. R. C. Kessler, W. T. Chiu, O. Demler, and E. E. Walters, "Prevalence, Severity, and Comorbidity of

Twelve-Month DSM-IV Disorders in the National Comorbidity Survey Replication (NCS-R)," *Archives of General Psychiatry* 62, no. 6 (June 2005): 617–627, referenced in The National Institute of Mental Health, "The Numbers Count: Mental Disorders in America," 2008, http://www.nimh.nih.gov/health/publications/the-numbers count-mental-disorders-in-america/index.shtml (accessed July 8, 2009).

2. U.S. Census Bureau, "Population Estimates by Demographic Characteristics. Table 2: Annual Estimates of the Population by Selected Age Groups and Sex for the United States: April 1, 2000 to July 1, 2004 (NC-EST2004-02)," Population Division, U.S. Census Bureau, June 9, 2005, http://www.census.gov/popest/national/asrh/, referenced in The National Institute of Mental Health, "The Numbers Count: Mental Disorders in America."

Chapter 8
Find Your Rest in God

1. Rich Bayer, "Benefits of Happiness," Upper Bay Counseling and Support Services, Inc., http://www.upperbay .org/DO%20NOT%20TOUCH%20-%20WEBSITE/articles/benefits%20of%20happiness.pdf (accessed January 8, 2015).

2. Ibid.

3. Ibid.

4. Mind/Body Medical Institute, "Mindfulness," http://www.mbmi.org/pages/wi_ms1aa.asp (accessed April 13, 2005).

5. W. F. Fry et al., *Make 'Em Laugh* (Palo Alto, CA; Science and Behavior Books, 1972).

6. Janice Norris, "Laughter Is Good Medicine," Health Is Wealth (blog), *The Sun Times*, March 23, 2011, http://www.thesuntimes.com/newsnow/x13293848/Laughter-is-good-medicine (accessed January 8, 2015).

7. University of Maryland Medical Center, "Laughter Is Good for Your Heart, According to a New University of Maryland Medical Center Study," news release, November 15, 2000, http://www.umm.edu/news/releases/laughter.htm (accessed January 8, 2015).

8. D. D. Danner, D. Snowden, and W. V. Friesen, "Positive Emotions in Early Life and Longevity: Findings From the Nun Study," *Journal of Personality and Social Psychology* 80 (2001): 804–813, referenced in Charles D. Kerns, "Gratitude at Work," *Graziadio Business Review* 9, no. 4 (2006), http://gbr.pepperdine.edu/064/quote/17764/ (accessed January 8, 2015).

9. QuotationsBook.com, http://www.quotationsbook.com/quote/17764/ (accessed January 8, 2015).

INDEX

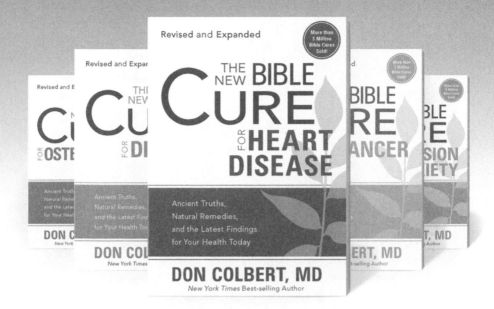

YOU WANT TO BE HEALTHY.
GOD WANTS YOU TO BE HEALTHY.

In each book of the Bible Cure series you will find helpful alternative medical information together with uplifting and faith-building biblical truths.

The New Bible Cure for Heart Disease
The New Bible Cure for Cancer
The New Bible Cure for Depression & Anxiety
The New Bible Cure for Osteoporosis
The New Bible Cure for Sleep Disorders
The New Bible Cure for Diabetes
The Bible Cure for ADD and Hyperactivity
The Bible Cure for Allergies
The Bible Cure for Arthritis
The Bible Cure for Asthma
The Bible Cure for Autoimmune Diseases
The Bible Cure for Back Pain
The Bible Cure for Candida and Yeast Infections
The Bible Cure for Chronic Fatigue & Fibromyalgia
The Bible Cure for Colds and Flu

The Bible Cure for Headaches
The Bible Cure for Heartburn and Indigestion
The Bible Cure for Hepatitis C
The Bible Cure for High Blood Pressure
The Bible Cure for High Cholesterol
The Bible Cure for Irritable Bowel Syndrome
The Bible Cure for Memory Loss
The Bible Cure for Menopause
The Bible Cure Recipes for Overcoming Candida
The Bible Cure for PMS & Mood Swings
The Bible Cure for Prostate Disorders
The Bible Cure for Skin Disorders
The Bible Cure for Stress
The Bible Cure for Thyroid Disorder
The Bible Cure for Weight Loss & Muscle Gain

NOW AVAILABLE AS E-BOOKS

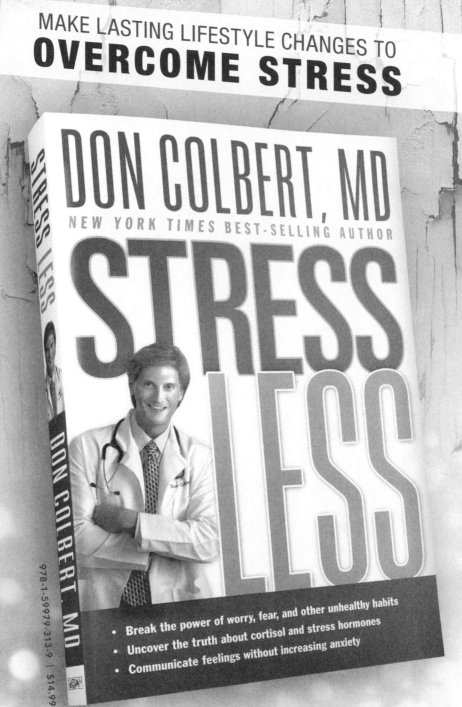